The Sisters' Story

PART TWO

SAINT MARYS HOSPITAL – MAYO CLINIC

1939 TO *1980*

The Sisters' Story

PART TWO

SAINT MARYS HOSPITAL – MAYO CLINIC

1939 TO *1980*

Sister Ellen Whelan, O.S.F.

Mayo Foundation for Medical Education and Research
Rochester, Minnesota 55905

Printed in the United States of America

5 4 3 2 1

Library of Congress Control Number: 2007928765

ISBN 13: 978-1-893005-99-0
ISBN 10: 1-893005-99-2

TABLE OF CONTENTS

FOREWORD

Like a reaper's blade, a great swath of epic events swept across the twentieth century, punctuated by two world wars with a worldwide economic depression. The pioneering Sisters of Saint Francis and the Mayo family were not immune to the scourge of those epic events (together they had established one of the preeminent hospitals in the United States in the latter part of the previous century). During the first half of the 1900s, crisis after crisis affected the hospital, its Sisters, and the growing staff of Mayo Clinic. The Franciscans and Mayos faced these critical challenges with a determined attitude and a cooperative spirit. Each crisis seemed to strengthen the two institutions—not weaken them. The crises brought with them new innovations and new ways of treating the sick—breakthroughs which would ultimately increase medical knowledge and make new therapeutic options available to the medical community.

This story, with its interwoven episodes, leaves one with an appreciation for the resolve and genius that characterized the Sisters of Saint Marys Hospital and the doctors of Mayo Clinic. Told in a narrative style that is easy to understand, Sister Ellen makes us feel as though we had a personal acquaintance with so many of the monumental figures that built the history of these two great organizations. One cannot but be humbled by the perseverance, the dedication to the patient, and the adherence to principles that these giants of health care exhibited. The servant leadership exhibited by the leaders of Saint Marys Hospital truly can be held up as a worthwhile example for the leaders of health care in the twenty-first century.

Craig Smoldt

Chair, Department of Facilities & Support Services
Rochester, Minnesota

FOREWORD

"An on-going challenge for Sisters, young and old alike," writes Sister Ellen Whelan, "was setting aside personal interests in service to the common good. The spirit of sacrifice, a striking characteristic of Saint Marys' Sisters, was essential in lives dedicated to serving others." The saga of the Sisters' story is an astounding drama of women *steeped in faith*, who were *anchored* in Mother Alfred's solemn belief that "obstacles were merely opportunities." The Sisters' extraordinary gifts of leadership and self-sacrifice were *guided* by the clarity of an inner vision that gave birth to the "miracle in a cornfield." This miracle is the life that became Saint Marys Hospital and Mayo Clinic.

In the decade of the 1930s, the Sisters were faced with daunting challenges that included the condemnation of the much-needed medical wing. Concurrently, a 40% drop in patient population, which affected revenues required to maintain the hospital, put the congregation at risk of bankruptcy. Then, World War II, and the country's call for nurses and doctors left Mayo and Saint Marys with critical staffing needs. Finally, perhaps the most difficult challenge was the shortage of Sisters available to serve at Saint Marys following the Second Vatican Council.

It was precisely in these moments of acute need that the selflessness and courage of the Sisters was most visible. Nothing was beyond the possibility of the Sisters and their Mayo partners who clearly recognized that their common purpose was the welfare of each patient. Dr. W. Eugene Mayberry said of the Sisters: "I believe it was the religious calling of the Sisters that made them such excellent colleagues for Mayo. Their lives were dedicated to the service of others and not to personal fame." Sister Ellen vividly captures the essence of this unique partnership, which placed the common good above every personal need. *The Sisters' Story, Part Two*, challenges its readers to search for ways that our world can be improved when the common good becomes the major focus of our shared efforts.

Sister Tierney Trueman, O.S.F.

President, Sisters of Saint Francis
Rochester, Minnesota

ACKNOWLEDGMENTS

Behind *The Sisters' Story, Part Two* is another story, a chronicle of colleagues, friends, and family whose support made the book a reality. Among them, my religious congregation, the Sisters of Saint Francis, who offered prayer, friendship, and financial resources. Jerry Mahoney and Jeanne Klein of the Saint Marys Hospital Sponsorship Board provided key assistance. Thanks to Jerry's efforts, generous donors contributed funds for publication costs. I'm most grateful to Mayo Administration, Saint Marys Hospital Auxiliary/Volunteers, and the Saint Marys Hospital Sponsorship Board for their financial help.

Gifted, knowledgeable, and invested readers provided me with important perspectives on each chapter and, ultimately, on the book overall. With warmest thanks to Franciscan Sisters Generose Gervais, Katarina Schuth, Lauren Weinandt, Marlene Pinzka, and Moira Tighe, along with Pamela O. Johnson, Stephen Kopecky, M.D., David Leonard, W. Eugene Mayberry, M.D., Donald McIlrath, M.D., Alice McIlrath, Judith Thistle, Tony Wiggins, and Rosemary Yaecker. Richard "Dick" Reitemeier, M.D., who died December 18, 2006, is remembered with deep respect and gratitude for his support and help.

Writing the book required consultation on a wide variety of subjects. Personal interviews offered insights on the human side of the story as well as important scientific and technical information. Sister Gavin Hagan's research efforts were particularly helpful, as were those of librarians and archivists at Mayo Clinic Libraries: Saint Marys Hospital Staff Library, Colonial Library, and the Plummer Library; the Mayo Historical Unit; Assisi Heights; the Rochester Public Library; and the History Center of Olmsted County.

The staff of several Mayo departments provided invaluable assistance throughout the process. My thanks to Communication Technology services for their generous help and patience. Production and publication of the book required a high degree of coordination and expertise by the staff of the Mayo Clinic Section of Scientific Publications, Publishing and Media

Technology Services, and Media Support Services. To these persons and to all who contributed to the project directly or indirectly, I offer thanks, not only for their help, but for their unfailing reminder that it is indeed more blessed to give than to receive.

Sister Ellen Whelan, O.S.F.

May 22, 2007

CHAPTER 1

Hospital Condemned

*I*n the spring of 1936, the middle of the Great Depression when Franklin Roosevelt was president, state Fire Marshal Henry George wrote Mayo Clinic a scathing letter condemning the medical wing of Saint Marys Hospital. "Rochester should lead in providing fireproof hospitals," he admonished them. "The fact that Rochester is known as the leading medical center of America makes it mandatory to provide the same high standard in the protection of persons who are their guests and patients from fire." Henry George's primary concern was the old medical wing of Saint Marys Hospital. The medical wing, however, was not Mayo property, but was owned and operated by the Sisters of Saint Francis of Rochester, Minnesota. Henry George's reason for writing to Mayo Clinic isn't clear. He may have thought the Sisters only managed the hospital; perhaps he didn't care to talk tough to women, let alone nuns.

Well before the fire marshal wrote his letter, Saint Marys' medical wing had been of concern to the Sisters. They had remodeled the building back in the 1920s, but those renovations, which were modest at best, were inadequate. The hospital needed a new medical wing. Finding funds to meet this need, however, seemed almost impossible. Like millions of others, the Sisters were caught in the iron grip of the Great Depression. Widespread, prolonged unemployment and loss of wages kept patients from coming to Rochester for treatment. By the early 1930s, hospital registrations declined by 40% and threatened to sink lower. Declining hospital revenues had serious consequences for the entire Franciscan congregation, as hospital earnings helped support the congregation's educational works. Of more

1

immediate importance, failure to make scheduled payments on large debts placed the Sisters of Saint Francis at risk for bankruptcy.

Condemnation of the medical building was potentially a lethal blow to the entire hospital. "The miracle in a cornfield," however, had a remarkable history of surviving enormous obstacles. Indeed, the genesis of Saint Marys Hospital in 1883, over 50 years earlier, was a natural disaster. A devastating tornado had leveled Rochester, and Mayor Samuel Whitten wired Governor Lucius F. Hubbard the following message: "Rochester is in ruins. Twenty-four people were killed. Over forty are seriously injured. One-third of the city laid waste. We need immediate help."

Rochester's leading physician, William Worrall Mayo, M.D., who headed emergency medical efforts, asked assistance from Mother Alfred Moes, mother superior of the local convent. She agreed readily and Sisters supervised a temporary hospital throughout the emergency. This experience

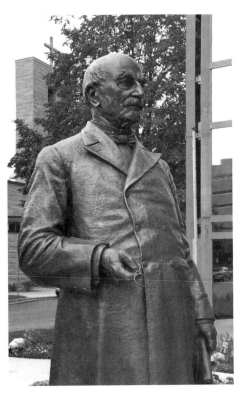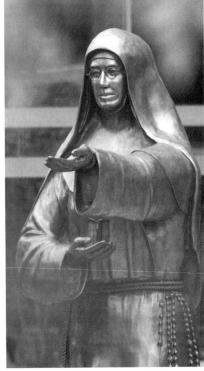

Founders William Worrall Mayo, M.D., and Mother Alfred Moes, Feith Family Statuary Park, Mayo Clinic, Rochester, Minnesota.

convinced Mother Alfred that Rochester needed a permanent hospital, and she approached Dr. W. W. Mayo with her idea. Dr. Mayo argued that the town was too small to support a hospital and reminded her that the public shunned them as "pest houses." Furthermore, it would be a costly undertaking with no assurance of success. In her indomitable way, Mother Alfred insisted she could build a hospital that would succeed and asked Dr. Mayo to take charge of it. To that end, through frugality and hard work, the Sisters raised enough money in 4 years for the project to begin. Dr. W. W. Mayo and Mother Alfred chose a site about a mile west of downtown and planned carefully for the new hospital.

Saint Marys Hospital opened on September 30, 1889, with 27 beds and two physicians, the sons of Dr. W. W. Mayo: 28-year-old William J. Mayo, M.D. (Dr. Will), with 6 years' experience and Charles H. Mayo, M.D. (Dr. Charlie), just out of medical school. At Mother Alfred's request, Dr. W. W. Mayo tried to organize a larger staff, but met with evasion and outright refusal. According to Mayo biographer Helen Clapesattle, the physicians he approached wanted no part of a venture that was sure to fail because of increasing anti-Catholicism and public fears of "black-robed nuns and a chapel for the practice of popery." Dr. W. W. Mayo, then 70 years old, recognized that the success of the new enterprise must rest on the shoulders of the two young Mayos. "The father became consulting physician and surgeon, and they the attending staff."

There were only four pioneer Sisters at Saint Marys at first, Sisters Sylvester Burke, Fidelis Cashion, Fabian Halloran, and Constantine Koupal. Three more arrived after the hospital opened, among them Sister Mary Joseph Dempsey (Sister Joseph), who would serve as superintendent for almost 50 years. Untrained as nurses, they learned the rudiments of the nursing profession from Edith Graham, Rochester's first graduate nurse, who later married Dr. Charlie. The partnership of the young Mayos and the Franciscan Sisters began tentatively. Indeed, at first glance, they appeared to have little in common. The Protestant Mayos, even in the small community of Rochester, were of a different social strata from the Sisters. The young men may have viewed the life of religious Sisters with some admiration, but it was clearly outside their experience. Their father's friendship with Mother Alfred and local priests made the Catholic religion less foreign and forbidding to them. Despite the diversity of their backgrounds, such mutual associations helped bridge their differences. Most importantly, they trusted each other's commitment to a common goal that transcended sectarian

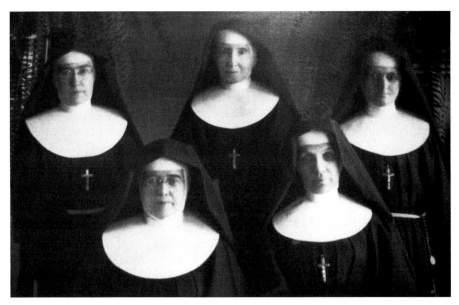

Pioneer Sisters of Saint Marys Hospital. Sisters Joseph Dempsey, Constantine Koupal (front row from left), Sylvester Burke, Fidelis Cashion, and Fabian Halloran (back row). (From Saint Marys Hospital Historical Display: More Than a Century of Caring. Rochester, MN: Mayo Press, 2001, p 4.)

belief—the service of suffering humanity. Success of the hospital, their over-riding goal, gave them courage and resourcefulness to overcome challenges.

Lack of funds was the Sisters' central problem when the hospital opened. They had no furnishings except for a dozen iron cots, a few dozen unbleached muslin sheets and pillowcases, and some rough gowns. Ill-fitting mattresses slipped around on the springs; just keeping the patient on the bed and the mattress on the springs was difficult. When eight patients came the first week, the Sisters gave up their own beds to make room for more patients. Regular duties demanded a rigorous schedule that began at 3:00 or 4:00 a.m. and ended at 11:00 p.m. or midnight. If a private nurse was needed at night, a Sister stayed up and remained on duty until the next night. Working 2 days and an intervening night was not unusual.

Demands on the Mayo brothers were equally rigorous. For the first 3 years there was no male orderly. On alternating nights, these young physicians took responsibility for nursing male patients who needed special attention. Sister Joseph later recalled the spirit of Saint Marys' nurses and doctors: "Their duty was to alleviate human suffering and to save human lives—and they did it."

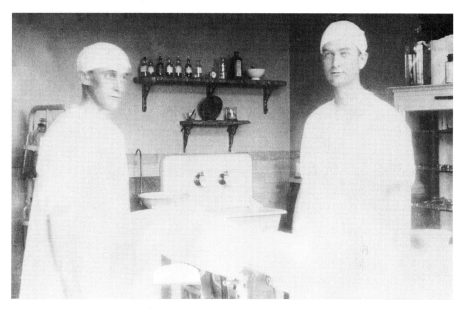

The young Doctors Mayo. (From Saint Marys Hospital Archives.)

The Franciscans and Mayos faced a critical challenge 3 years after the hospital opened. A rival physician, W. A. Allen, M.D., built a competing hospital that offered an alternative to one owned by Catholic Sisters. Some local Protestants welcomed Riverside Hospital as one they could use "without doing outrage to their convictions by furthering an agency of the hated and alien Catholic Church."

When asked to attend patients at Riverside Hospital, the Mayos realized that their refusal would make them a target of abuse by their fellow Protestants. However, dividing their practice would have disastrous consequences for Saint Marys, because most of their patients would choose the non-Catholic hospital. Mayo biographer Helen Clapesattle assessed their decision: ". . . the Mayos were wise enough to see the advantages of centralizing their practice in one hospital, under one staff—particularly a hospital and staff they controlled . . . moreover, the Mayos felt a strong moral obligation to the Sisters of Saint Francis . . . And finally, the Mayos were not men inclined to knuckle under to the public clamor or the pressure of opposition." Their decision to serve only patients at Saint Marys brought highly emotional censure and criticism from a segment of the Protestant population. In response, the Mayos quietly focused on their practice and cared for patients. When critics attacked them and waited for a reply, they chose to ignore the abuse and appeared unperturbed by it.

Riverside Hospital had operated successfully for over 2 years when Dr. Allen, for unknown reasons, announced he was moving to St. Paul, Minnesota. Riverside Hospital closed and sold its beds and other movables to Saint Marys Hospital.

The Sisters' records give no account of their response to the events that threatened Saint Marys Hospital. Presumably, it was an extraordinarily difficult time for them, because they were powerless to do anything about pervasive anti-Catholicism. They wanted their hospital to succeed, but, in truth, believed the success of Saint Marys was not up to them, but was in God's hands. And so, as was their custom in times of difficulty and decision, they fasted and prayed that God would bless the work of their hands.

Undoubtedly the Sisters were grateful for the unexpected departure of Dr. Allen and the subsequent closing of Riverside Hospital. Their overwhelming gratitude and admiration, however, went to the Mayos. They would never forget how the Mayos endured public abuse with steadfast courage on their behalf; the Mayos' unswerving loyalty had almost certainly saved the hospital. The strident controversy surrounding Riverside Hospital cemented the relationship between the Doctors Mayo and the Sisters at Saint Marys Hospital. Despite inexperience, hardship, and hostility, they had learned to depend on each other.

Sister Joseph, as Dr. Will's first assistant in surgery, was well aware of the gracious providence that opened the hospital in 1889, as a new era of surgery began. Infection was a surgeon's greatest nemesis and the reason for the public's fear of hospitals. Even after successful surgical procedures, septic infections invaded the patient's wounds and caused high fever and, many times, death. Scottish surgeon Joseph Lister, in 1867, demonstrated that bacterial microorganisms caused surgical infections and that antisepsis could kill them. The Mayos incorporated Lister's technique, wet antisepsis, in their surgery with astonishing results: of the 1,037 patents admitted in the first 2 years, patient deaths numbered only 22. Patients went home cured and, in turn, told others about their experience. Such a low mortality rate, which brought recognition for the abilities of the Doctors Mayo, also brought increasing numbers of patients to Saint Marys Hospital.

The Mayos continued to keep pace with new developments in surgery. One at a time, over the next years, they made extended visits to leading medical centers and observed the work of selected surgeons. They brought back new ideas and shared them with the Sisters, who were as committed to improving in their areas of practice as the Mayos were in surgery. Working in their remote location, far from urban centers and nearby competitors, the Mayos performed some operations by the hundreds, and even by the thousands. According to a surgeon colleague, the articles they contributed to medical journals, which described their successes in unprecedented numbers of cases, sent the Mayo Clinic soaring into worldwide prominence during the years 1895 to 1906. Indeed, by 1906 the Mayo surgeons had performed over 5,000 operations, more than any hospital in the United States.

Unprecedented growth created problems of overcrowding and prompted the Mayos to begin a series of requests for hospital additions. By 1912, five new additions increased the hospital's capacity to 300 beds and six operating rooms. It bears noting that these Mayo initiatives and the Sisters' response characterized their interaction on building improvement for the next hundred years. Typically, physicians explained the need for a new addition and presented a well-conceived building plan. After discussion and adjustments, when necessary, the Sisters committed resources and the building went forward. On the hospital's silver anniversary, in 1914, Saint Marys was treating almost 8,000 inpatients per year and nearly 2,000 outpatients.

With the hospital's success came significant earnings. From the beginning, these earnings, whenever possible, went back into the institution. The Mayos, particularly Dr. Will, were relieved when the hospital began paying its own way. They wanted Saint Marys to become fully self-supporting. In their view, the hospital should earn enough money for its own charities, as they did, and finance its own improvements. The Mayos adopted the policy of telling patients to pay the Sisters' bill first and their bill for professional services second. Around the time of the hospital's silver anniversary, the Sisters bought land in anticipation of Mayo requests for future buildings. They also purchased a 200-acre farm to provide patients with fresh food of high quality and signed $2,225,000 in contracts for construction of a new surgical pavilion, later named the Joseph Building in honor of Sister Joseph.

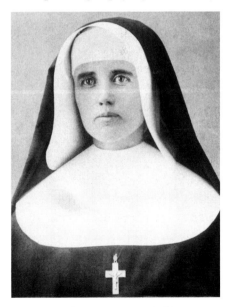

Sister Joseph Dempsey, 1890. (From Saint Marys Hospital Archives.)

The year 1914, with the dedication of its first clinical building, was a milestone for Mayo Clinic. After decades of renting office space, the Doctors Mayo asked Henry S. Plummer, M.D., to design a clinic structure that would house the medical practice, educational facilities, and research laboratories under one roof. The structure, later simply called the 1914 Building, stood on the original site of Dr. W. W. Mayo's home in downtown Rochester. Subsequently, the Mayos took several important institutional initiatives.

Early on, the Mayos' growing practice prompted them to ask other physicians, like Dr. Plummer, to join them. These physicians were selected carefully; their talents in medical and laboratory specialties complemented the Mayos' surgical skills and brought a new dimension to patient services. The Mayos long believed that the advantages of medical specialization could be achieved only if specialists functioned as a unit in relation to the patient. "A sick man is not like a wagon to be taken apart and repaired in pieces; he must be examined and treated as a whole."

Dr. Plummer formulated an organizational plan that integrated all the activities of the medical practice, which included education and research. February 18, 1915, the Mayos signed incorporation papers creating a new entity, Mayo Foundation for Medical Education and Research. The brothers solidified their commitment with an endowment to the Foundation of $1.5 million of their own savings, as well as all the physical properties and assets of the Clinic.

According to the Foundation agreement, ". . . the Mayos, their partners, and all future Mayo physicians would receive a salary and not profit personally from the proceeds of the practice. All proceeds beyond operating expenses were henceforth contributed to education, research, and patient care." This was a bold step and ensured that Mayo Clinic would survive its founders' retirements and deaths. From this initiative, Mayo Clinic emerged as a distinct institution and a new model of private group practice.

The Sisters faced a new reality when Mayo Clinic became a separate institution. Mutual trust forged in their first 25 years, however, bonded them personally and institutionally. Determined to continue the partnership, the Franciscans spared no effort or financial investment to attain that end and believed their extensive property acquisitions would meet future Clinic needs. Unfortunately, the Great Depression would prove the Sisters wrong.

The Depression wreaked financial havoc for Mayo Clinic as well as Saint Marys Hospital. Chief administrator Harry J. Harwick described the early thirties as "unquestionably the most difficult" of his 44 years with

Mayo. Registration figures "dropped and dropped and kept on dropping—from 79,000 in 1929 to less than 50,000 in 1932." Mayo Clinic borrowed money to meet payrolls and implemented drastic action to reduce operating costs. Harwick reflected, "Most bitter of all, the most difficult of my life, was the decision to go to the Mayo Board and recommend that the salaries of all Clinic staffs be cut to the bone. I made this recommendation with the full knowledge that many cherished plans of Clinic families would be altered or ended entirely. If the Clinic and the community were to weather this storm at all there was no alternative. For the first time in my life, I knew what it was to go to bed, but not to sleep."

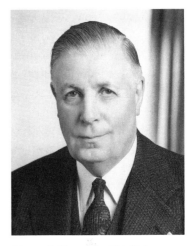

Harry J. Harwick, Chief Mayo Administrator, 1908-1952.

The Board of Governors concurred with the recommendation and on January 5, 1932, voted in favor of a comprehensive reduction of salaries, shown in Table 1.

Table 1. Mayo Clinic Salary Reductions Implemented During the Great Depression*†

Reduction for professional staff	
Salary under $5,000	15%
Salary between $5,000 and $10,000	20%
Salary between $10,000 and $15,000	25%
Salary between $15,000 and $20,000	30%
Salary over $20,000	35%
Stipends for surgical and clinical assistants	
First-year, $800	
Second-year, $900	
Third-year, $1,000	
Fourth-year, $1,200	
Fifth-year, $1,500	

*Nonprofessional employees, in whatever departments possible, to be placed on a 4.5-day week instead of a 5.5-day week, the day off to be at the expense of the employee.

†The per diem travelling allowance for all members of the Mayo Clinic staff reduced to $7.00 per day plus railroad and Pullman fares.

Many patients, unable to supply their families with basic needs, were unable to pay their medical bills. Harry J. Harwick, Mayo Clinic administrator, noted that some organizations introduced tough collection policies, but not Mayo Clinic. Indeed, at Dr. Will's suggestion, the Board of Governors adopted an even more lenient collection policy than that held before the Depression. "When it has been quite well demonstrated than an account is uncollectible, it is better to write the patient a pleasant letter enclosing a receipted bill, rather than engaging in any controversy or attempting to press collection indefinitely."

Dr. Will's words to the Board recall the spirit of his father, who taught his sons by example: "Our father recognized certain definite social obligations. He believed that any man who had better opportunity than others, greater strength of mind, body, or character owed something to those who had not been so provided." Dr. W. W. Mayo didn't collect fees from persons who were "down on their luck." He wouldn't take money "from a struggling widow or a farmer with a load of debt" and refused to accept a mortgage in payment or sue for an account.

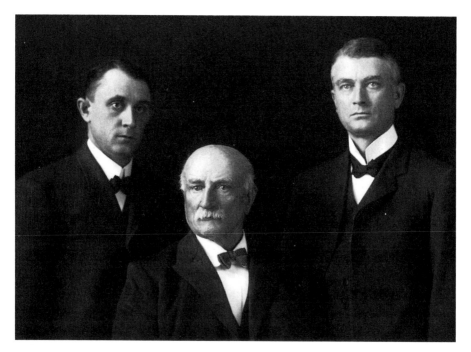

William Worrall Mayo, M.D. (center), and his sons, Charles H. Mayo, M.D. (left), and William J. Mayo, M.D. (right), around 1900.

It was during this difficult time of the Great Depression that the Board of Governors received the Minnesota State fire marshal's letter noted earlier, which condemned Saint Marys' medical wing on March 11, 1936. Patient safety and the Clinic's reputation were of grave concern and required immediate action. Eschewing protocol, the Board of Governors wrote directly to the Franciscan mother superior, Mother Aquinas Norton. Their letter, delivered by courier to her offices a few blocks away, quickly came to the point. In summary, they wrote that the state fire marshal's condemnation of the medical wing was a matter of public record. The Clinic had a moral obligation to safeguard patients against injury by fire. Such injuries could find the hospital guilty of gross negligence and prejudice patients from coming to Rochester. Confident that the Sisters were equally concerned, the Board recommended an early meeting of the Saint Marys Hospital Committee as, "the best opportunity for candid and sympathetic discussion and effecting a program to remedy the existing conditions." Perhaps, to reassure Mother Aquinas of their good will, the letter mentioned two hospital committee members highly regarded by the Sisters, chief of surgery, Melvin S. Henderson, M.D., and Mayo Clinic administrator, Harry Harwick.

Mother Aquinas responded immediately; within 2 weeks, Dr. Henderson reported several meetings with her, as did Harry Harwick. Later in the year, Donald C. Balfour, M.D., chair of the Board of Governors, reported that Saint Marys was considering "the building of a new medical unit west of the present surgical unit." The following February he was more specific: "The Sisters of Saint Francis are planning a 235-bed hospital addition immediately west of the present surgical pavilion to be used as a medical wing." Construction of the building would begin in 2 years.

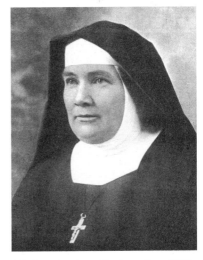

The Great Depression ended, by most standards, in 1939. During the decade of the thirties, in the face of enormous financial burdens, Mayo leaders and their colleagues had successfully kept the institution intact. Harry Harwick later called the Depression, "the most unifying influence" in all of the Clinic's history. "In this adversity members of all staffs [sic] pulled together to see the thing through.

Mother Aquinas Norton, circa 1933.

Adversity, at any time, if faced up to and beaten, is not at all a bad thing: among other rewards, one gains in wisdom for the very good reason that one must if one is to survive."

Wisdom expressed in teamwork, mutual trust, and interdependence stood the Clinic in good stead when they faced their greatest losses, the deaths of their beloved founders. At the height of their careers, 20 years earlier, the Mayos began grooming their successors and developing an organizational plan. They established a Board of Governors charged with operating the Clinic and instituted a system of committees responsible for specific areas within the Clinic. Committees, whose members came primarily from the medical staff, reported regularly to the Board on their actions and deliberations. Through committee activities, members learned about Clinic operations and later became candidates for appointment to the Board of Governors.

In 1939, the Doctors Mayo died within 2 months of each other. Dr. Charles H. Mayo, 73 years old, died of lobar pneumonia on May 26, in Chicago, Illinois. Dr. William J. Mayo, 78 years old, died in his sleep in Rochester on July 28. According to Harwick, the years following the Mayos' deaths, "were the period of greatest danger to the institution. Had the staffs [sic] wavered, become fearful or split into cliques, the Clinic might indeed have been in serious trouble. Happily, this was not the case. Instead, as they had in the Depression, the staffs [sic] drew closer together to face this new challenge." For the Sisters at Saint Marys Hospital, the death of the beloved and trusted brothers was a deep personal loss. In addition, the reality of Mayo Clinic's new leadership, without the Doctors Mayo at the helm, created concern for the future of the hospital.

At this time of transition, during the Great Depression, the Franciscan congregation was fortunate to have Mother Aquinas Norton as mother superior. Experience in business and finance, along with a strong academic background, were among her valuable assets. Before joining the Franciscans, she pursued business studies in college, helped her father run the family lumber business, and later went to the College of Saint Teresa in Winona, Minnesota, for her baccalaureate degree. After entering the congregation, superiors assigned her to teach at the College of Saint Teresa and she went on for further study. She earned a Master of Arts degree from the University of Minnesota and a Ph.D. degree in history from Catholic University of America in Washington, DC. Perhaps Mother Aquinas's greatest personal asset as congregational leader was an ability to assess complex problems and enlist help from others for their solution. She took the lead on the medical wing project and, for 3 years (1936-1939), tenaciously sought assistance for building the addition. In the process, Mother Aquinas tapped a wide array of resources, from banks and investors in Chicago and Milwaukee, to the pope and Vatican officials in Rome, to the Franciscan saint, Anthony of Padua, reputedly the finder of lost items, including money.

Mother Aquinas's first order of business was to extricate the Congregation from threatened bankruptcy. Loans totaling $5 million for building projects at the College of Saint Teresa came due about the same time she took office in 1934. Indeed, the day after her installation, the sheriff informed her that the congregation faced bankruptcy for failing to make payments on their large debt. Unknown to Mother Aquinas, the congregation's business agent in Chicago, charged with the debt repayment, kept $350,000 of the Sisters' payments for himself. Mother Aquinas immediately appointed Sister Adele O'Neil congregational treasurer. Young, lively, and petite, Sister Adele possessed disarming financial expertise and dogged determination. Like Mother Aquinas, she also had learned about finance from working with her family's business before entering the congregation.

Mother Aquinas asked the bishop of Winona, Minnesota, Francis M. Kelly, and his financial advisors to meet with her about the financial crisis. To their surprise, the diminutive Sister Adele spoke up and suggested that she serve as business agent rather than paying a large commission. Given the desperate situation, they agreed. Later, Sister Adele told the astonishing story of how she, with Sister Rita Rishavy's help, repaid the noteholders and "no one lost a dollar of principal." Eighty percent of the creditors were people from Chicago. As Sister Adele put it, "we made friends with the Continental Bank of Chicago and found the vice president very helpful." He gave them regular use of a conference room with telephone and typewriter. About once a week, the two Sisters, with money from hospital receipts, took the night train to Chicago, where they worked all the next day repaying some creditors and calling on others to renew notes at a lower interest rate. Returning to Rochester

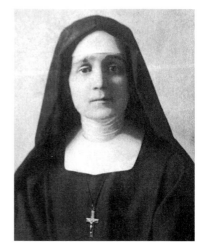

Sister Adele O'Neil, the Franciscans' remarkable young business agent. (From Assisi Heights Archives, Rochester, MN.)

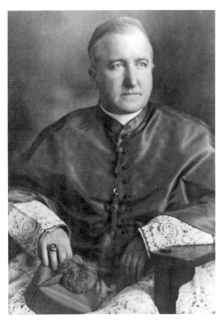

Bishop Francis M. Kelly, circa 1930. (Courtesy of the Diocese of Winona, Winona, MN. Used with permission.)

on the night train, they went directly to the motherhouse, where they wrote confirmation letters, often working until midnight without benefit of any office machines except their manual typewriter.

Re-establishing the congregation's credit appears to have taken Sister Adele the better part of 1936 and 1937. In the same timeframe, Mother Aquinas engaged an architectural firm and planned the new medical wing, at a projected cost of 2 million dollars. In the spring of 1938, she took an unprecedented step and enlisted help from the entire congregation. Mother Aquinas wrote every convent to ask each Sister for her participation in a prayer of petition, commonly called a novena. On Tuesdays from April 12 to June 7, Sisters prayed for Saint Anthony's intercession in finding a benefactor for the medical wing. In addition, Mother Aquinas asked each Sister "who feels she can fast on each of the nine Tuesdays without detriment to her health or work, please do so for this intention, if she is willing. All things are accomplished by prayer and fasting. God knows our difficulty and our need in this problem that is confronting our Congregation. He will not turn a deaf ear to our earnest, sincere, and fervent petitions."

Mother Aquinas's letter went to women already well instructed in prayer and sacrifice. Whether they served in schools or hospitals, the Great Depression taught them powerful lessons about the providence of God. About 400 of the congregation's 600 members were in education, typically teaching in diocesan rural school across the Midwest. Hard hit by the Depression, local parishes frequently couldn't pay the small stipend that provided heat for the convent and food for their table. When they could, local parishioners gave food to the Sisters out of their own meager supplies. Sisters pleaded with pastors for partial stipends, sometimes with no response. Harsh Minnesota winters without fuel and food forced Sisters to close some schools, at least temporarily. More often, they lowered the heat, ate the bare necessities, and kept the schools open. At Saint Marys Hospital, because of patient needs, Sisters suffered less from lack of heat and food. Lack of finances, however, forced them to reduce lay staff and their duties, already excessive, increased during the 1930s. As often happens, the Sisters' prayers were answered, but not quite as requested. While no benefactor appeared to give money for the medical wing, Mother Aquinas negotiated loans on good terms with banks in Chicago and Milwaukee. Further, Sister Adele reported that the Continental Bank in Chicago made their loan without a commitment fee and when she asked former noteholders for loans, almost all reinvested.

As a Catholic institution, Saint Marys Hospital had certain rights and obligations: one of them was a financial review of major building projects by Church hierarchy. Permission to build Saint Marys' medical wing required review by the local bishop, the cardinal in Washington, DC, and the pope in Rome. These churchmen and their advisors studied the congregation's substantive institutional report, submitted in Latin and English, carefully. Mother Aquinas's well-crafted report included a history of the hospital with explanation of the relationship with Mayo Clinic and an analysis of congregational finances and detailed plan for financing the project. In February of 1938, Mother Aquinas began a year of correspondence with Bishop Kelly in Winona, Cardinal Cicognani in Washington, DC, and Pope Pius XI in Rome. Their letters convey respect and concern for the congregation along with helpful guidance. In February of the following year, Cardinal Cicognani informed Mother Aquinas, in Latin and English, that the pope had approved the congregation's request. Graciously, he asked her not to pay the usual fee for the review—he had already written Rome for a reduction.

Mother Aquinas worked closely with Sister Joseph on plans for the medical wing. Most likely, it was this contact that prompted her to speak with her leadership council about Sister Joseph: "The General Superior suggested that it may be necessary in the near future, because of the failing health of Sister Mary Joseph, to appoint a new superintendent for Saint Mary's Hospital." Sister Domitilla DuRocher from Saint Marys Hospital was part of the council of four Franciscans elected to assist Mother Aquinas in congregational leadership. Sister Domitilla, then director of Saint Marys School of Nursing, was a national leader in her field and a natural successor to Sister Joseph. In 1937, Sister Domitilla became assistant administrator and assumed most of Sister Joseph's responsibilities, though not her title, until the latter's death on March 29, 1939.

Sister Joseph was already a legend before her death. She had received countless accolades, but praise made her uncomfortable. Typically she deflected compliments by praising others. If asked about her deep religious faith and uncommon kindness, she quickly credited her parents and their example. When recognized for achievements, she pointed to the unstinting service of all the Sisters at Saint Marys Hospital. Sister Joseph, a first-generation Irish-American, was a woman of fierce loyalty to her faith, her family, and her institution, in that order. As an institutional leader, she preferred to use a velvet glove, but this diminutive leader had no difficulty in claiming her authority. When questioned, she took a step back, fixed her challenger with the gaze of bright, brown eyes, and asked, "Who's running this institution?"

Stories about Sister Joseph's skills abounded from young surgeons who trained under Dr. Will when Sister Joseph was his first assistant. Such a person was Raymond P. Sullivan, M.D. (Sully), who became a distinguished surgeon in New York City. Much later, he told a Mayo audience about performing surgery with Dr. Will and Sister Joseph before a gallery of visiting physicians: "While working in Room 2 with Dr. Mayo, we had one case in which Dr. Braasch [W. F. Braasch, M.D.] had made a diagnosis of a stone in the right ureter. The patient was a very heavy man and Dr. Will made the usual attempt to locate the ureter and worked for quite a while until one point, when my arm from retraction was about paralyzed, Sister Joseph said, 'Will, you talk to them and Sully and I will go for it.' So Dr. Will stepped aside and in about three to five minutes, those wonderful little hands were in that wound and she said, 'Sully, just feel this,' and I said, 'What the hell, that feels like a stone.' She said, 'Here it is, Will,' and Dr. Mayo immediately located it, got it out, and Dr. Braasch was then very much delighted by the finding and Dr. Will turned around and told the audience, 'See what it means to have teamwork?'"

The Alumni Association of Mayo Foundation commissioned a bronze bust of Sister Joseph. The statue was unveiled at a memorial service for Sister Joseph, part of the hospital's Golden Anniversary celebration in 1939. Dr. Melvin Henderson paid her this tribute: "Her spirit is certainly with us, for here is where her heart lived. I shall always think of Sister Mary Joseph first in the role of surgical assistant where she worked for many years across the operating table from Dr. Will. Secondly, as a teacher, for she instructed

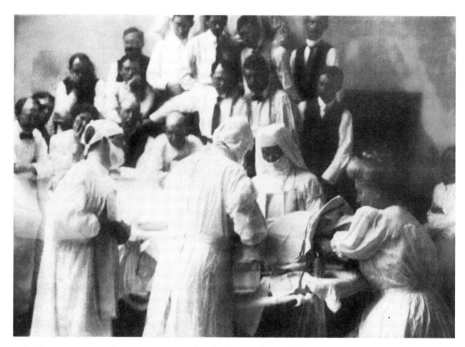

Visiting surgeons observe an operation being performed by William J. Mayo, M.D., assisted by Sister Joseph. (From Saint Marys Hospital Archives.)

not only nurses but doctors, and many of her students, 'her boys,' as she called them, are here today. Third, as administrator, for under her guidance the hospital was run quietly and efficiently. Sister Joseph was a model for all of us, who were oncoming surgeons in those days as we saw her stand erect and poised for action opposite our chief. She was keen eyed, quick as a flash, her small deft hands made no lost motion as she worked with absolute coordination with the surgeon. It was my position thirty years ago to be one of the surgical team of which Sister Joseph was a part and she taught me many things that have been of great value to me in my surgical career. . . . Because of the esteem, love, and affection which the staff of the Mayo Clinic had for this remarkable woman, our teacher, fellow administrator, and co-worker, we present to the Sisters of Saint Francis, this sculptured bust of Sister Mary Joseph."

The deaths of Doctors Will and Charlie and Sister Joseph in 1939, within five months of each other, ended the founding years of Saint Marys Hospital. Their story, striking in its own time and for future generations, suggests the presence of miracles in the ordinary happenings of human

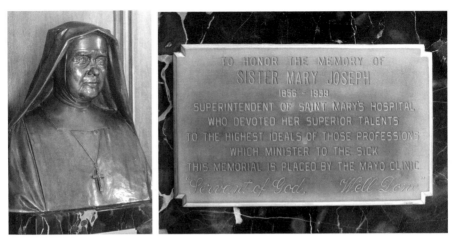

Bronze bust of Sister Mary Joseph Dempsey, 1939. A gift of the Alumni Association of the Mayo Foundation to Saint Marys Hospital, bearing the inscription, "Servant of God, Well Done."

relationships. Saint Marys was the only hospital in America, perhaps in the world, owned by Catholic Sisters in an exclusive partnership with nonsectarian physicians. Even more unusual, a handshake sealed this partnership for almost 100 years. The bronze bust of Sister Joseph bears an inscription that might be made of every Sister at Saint Marys Hospital:

"Servant of God, Well Done."

ENDNOTES

Page 1   **Mayo Clinic Board of Governors' Meeting Minutes, March 11, 1936.**
Minnesota fire marshal's letter.

Page 2   **Hodgson HW: *Rochester: City of the Prairie*. Northridge, CA: Windsor Publications, 1989, pp 25-26.**
Telegram from Rochester Mayor Samuel Whitten to Governor Lucius F. Hubbard.

Kraman C: *Odyssey in Faith: The Story of Mother Alfred Moes*. Rochester, MN: Sisters of Saint Francis, Assisi Heights, 1990, pp 1-7, 168.

Clapesattle H: *The Doctors Mayo*. Minneapolis: The University of Minnesota Press, 1941, pp 242-244.
The tornado in Rochester.

Page 3   **Kraman (pp 169-170).**

Clapesattle (p 246) describes how Mother Alfred approached Dr. W. W. Mayo about building a hospital.

Clapesattle (p 253) describes Dr. W. W. Mayo's attempt to recruit doctors.

Clapesattle (p 256) comments on the Doctors Mayo in new roles.

Page 4   **Saint Marys Hospital Annals.**
Sister Joseph Dempsey wrote a narrative about the early days of the hospital as an introduction to Saint Marys Hospital Annals.

Whelan E: *The Sisters' Story: Saint Marys Hospital—Mayo Clinic 1889-1939*. Rochester, MN: Mayo Foundation for Medical Education and Research, 2002, p 63.

Page 5   **Clapesattle (pp 264-267, 783).**
The story of the Riverside Hospital with bibliographic note.

Page 6   **Whelan (pp 72-73).**

Bordley J III, Harvey AM: *Two Centuries of American Medicine: 1776-1976*. Philadelphia: W. B. Saunders Company, 1976, pp 300-301.

Pages 6-7   Saint Marys Hospital Annals documents the surgical numbers.

Page 7   **Whelan E:** *The Sisters' Story: Saint Marys Hospital—Mayo Clinic 1889-1939*, **pp 81-82, 89-90.**

               A Century of Caring: 1889-1989. **Rochester, MN: Saint Marys Hospital, 1988, pp 29, 32.**
               Summarizes hospital admissions and building additions from 1889 to 1914.

Page 8   **Nelson CW:** *Mayo Roots: Profiling the Origins of Mayo Clinic.* **Rochester, MN: Mayo Historical Unit, Mayo Foundation, 1990, pp 116-117.**

               Mayo WJ: The Necessity of Cooperation in the Practice of Medicine. Rush Medical College Commencement Address. In: *Collected Papers of St. Mary's Hospital Proceedings of the Staff Meetings of the Mayo Clinic.* **Philadelphia: W. B. Saunders Company, 1910, pp 557-566.**

               Whelan (pp 106-107).

Page 8-9   **Harwick HJ:** *Forty-Four Years With the Mayo Clinic: 1908-1952.* **Rochester, MN: Whiting Press, 1957, pp 28-29.**

Page 9   **Mayo Clinic Board of Governors' Meeting Minutes, January 5, 1932.**
               Reduction in salaries and accompanying decisions.

Page 10   **Mayo Clinic Board of Governors' Meeting Minutes, October 21, 1931.**
               Dr. W. J. Mayo's recommendation on collection policy.

               Clapesattle H: *The Doctors Mayo*, **p 179.**
               Quote from Dr. W. J. Mayo.

               Clapesattle (p 152) references Dr. W. W. Mayo's collection policies.

Page 11   **Mayo Clinic Board of Governors' Meeting Minutes, March 11, 1936.**
               Letter from the state fire marshal and Board of Governors' letter to Mother Aquinas.

               Mayo Clinic Board of Governors' Meeting Minutes, March 18, 1936 and March 27, 1936.
               Dr. Henderson's and Mr. Harwick's references to meetings with Mother Aquinas.

Mayo Clinic Board of Governors' Meeting Minutes, November 4, 1936 and February 3, 1937.
Dr. Balfour's references to Saint Marys Hospital's proposed medical wing.

Pages 11-12   **Harwick HJ:** *Forty-Four Years With the Mayo Clinic: 1908-1952,* **p 30.**

Page 12   **Harwick (pp 32-33).**

Page 13   Taped interview with Sister M. Adele O'Neil, February 29, 1980.

Whelan E: *The Sisters' Story: Saint Marys Hospital—Mayo Clinic 1889-1939,* **pp 142-143.**

Page 14   **Sisters of Saint Francis General Council Meeting Minutes, March 26, 1938.**
Letter from Mother Aquinas to all convents.

Page 15   **Sisters of Saint Francis General Council Meeting Minutes, December 8, 1937.**
Mother Aquinas' remarks about Sister Joseph Dempsey.

Page 16   **Homan MC:** *Years of Vision, 1903-1928: A History of the Sisters of the Third Order Regular of Saint Francis of the Congregation of Our Lady of Lourdes, Rochester, Minnesota.* **Unpublished Masters Thesis, Catholic University of America, Washington, DC, 1956, pp 102, 115.**
Some of the Sister Joseph's characteristics noted.

Whelan (pp 97-98).

Transcription of a tape recording made in October, 1961 at Rochester, Minnesota by Dr. Raymond P. Sullivan, 14 E. 75th Street, New York 21, NY.
Archives of the Mayo Historical Suite provided this reference and other information about Dr. Raymond P. Sullivan. A distinguished surgeon in New York City, Dr. Sullivan was Director of Surgery Emeritus at Saint Vincent's Hospital at the time of his death in 1963. An article in "Mayovox," October 27, 1962, describes him as "busy, bubbling with humor, a reminiscent gold mine of stories on the early days hereabouts." "It's said by those who knew both men well that Dr. Will, something of an austere man, relaxed more the "Sully" than with any other physician."

Page 17   **Mayo Clinic Board of Governors' Meeting Minutes, May 10, 1939.**
Reference to commissioning of bronze bust of Sister Joseph.

Saint Marys Alumnae Quarterly Vol. XXIV, no. 1, January 1940, pp 4-5.

Memorial Program, Saint Mary's Auditorium, Wednesday, October 25, 1939.
Dr. Henderson's remarks.

CHAPTER 2

Building for the Future

The superintendent of Saint Marys Hospital that succeeded Sister Mary Joseph Dempsey had impressive credentials—an Ivy League education and a distinguished reputation in nursing education. Sister Domitilla DuRocher assumed her new position with confidence and quickly grasped the hospital's needs. She built new structures on Saint Marys' strong foundation: a legacy from the pioneer Sisters. Those structures, some in concrete and others organizational, brought sweeping initiatives to every area of the institution, from building the medical wing to the creation of new departments. In a decade of hospital leadership, her achievements contributed immeasurably to the field of health care, not only to Saint Marys Hospital but also as models for hospitals across the country.

Though prodigious in her administrative accomplishments, Sister Domitilla's greatest contribution was

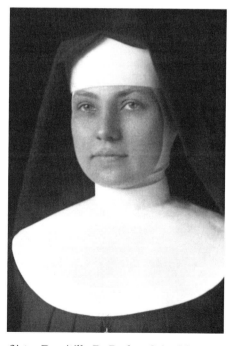

Sister Domitilla DuRocher, Saint Marys Hospital Administrator, 1939-1949. (From Assisi Heights Archives, Rochester, MN.)

23

to nursing. She and her indomitable colleagues, secular and religious, raised nursing from a disdained menial job to the status of a respected profession.

Sister Domitilla's service at Saint Marys Hospital spanned 40 years. Her story is all the more interesting for the enigmatic qualities of the woman herself. Lillian DuRocher, who would take the name Sister Domitilla, learned responsibility and initiative at an early age. The second oldest of 10 children, she grew up on a farm near Monroe, Michigan. Her parents, LaCombe and Josephine DuRocher, were of French descent with American ancestry that went back to 1708. Lillian inherited a subtle sense of humor and business acumen from her father. "From her mother, Lillian inherited a love for beauty and quiet and a deep religious nature." Josephine DuRocher inspired her daughter's devotion to St. Francis of Assisi. She read aloud to the family from a French edition of his life that stressed the saint's love for the poor and graciousness to lepers, "the poorest of the poor."

When Lillian was about to begin her senior year in high school, she made an unusual choice that illustrates her initiative and sense of purpose. One evening, through the stovepipe in her room, she overheard her father talking with his good friend, the superintendent of schools. They discussed the shortage of teachers for rural schools. When the superintendent asked if Lillian could take one of the positions, her father insisted, "She must finish high school first." The next morning, Lillian went to the superintendent, volunteered her services, and told her parents in the evening that she had signed a contract to teach. Astonished, they reluctantly gave permission; Lillian taught in rural schools for 3 years until joining the Rochester Franciscans in 1910.

Sister Domitilla finished high school as a Franciscan novice and taught in parochial schools for 3 years. When the mother superior appealed for nurses in 1916, she entered Saint Marys School of Nursing and excelled in her studies. According to Sister Mary Brigh Cassidy, she was "an outstanding student, not in a brilliant, flashy manner but in thorough-going performance, complete understanding, and utter reliability. Sister Domitilla never left a problem until she had thoroughly mastered it." Sister Joseph also recognized Sister Domitilla's gifts and asked her to direct Saint Marys School of Nursing, the first Sister to head the school since its founding in 1906. To prepare for the assignment, she entered Columbia University, Teachers College, Department of Nursing and Health in the fall of 1918, only a few months after receiving her nursing diploma. The department, affectionately called "the motherhouse," was the pioneer degree program in nursing; Sister Domitilla was the first American Sister to receive a degree in nursing.

World War I ended in November of 1918, about the same time that Sister Domitilla entered Columbia. An event of such worldwide proportion precipitated social and economic change and brought important new opportunities for American women. Passage of the Nineteenth Amendment to the Constitution of the United States gave women the right to vote. Nurses were among the advocates for women's suffrage. With their sisters in arms, they labored 75 years for this achievement. Indeed, nursing history closely parallels the women's movement in America.

Like the entire nation, Sister Domitilla was caught up in the change and opportunity that were sweeping the country. When she entered Columbia she was 30 years old, from a parochial background, and just out of nursing school. She entered a major university whose faculty and graduates would help define the role of nursing. Her university experience and association with faculty and students made a lasting impact. The academic background she received as educational director and instructor in the basic sciences was invaluable. Friends made during these years invited her to join state and national nursing committees. Her contributions to nursing in this broader arena soon brought national recognition.

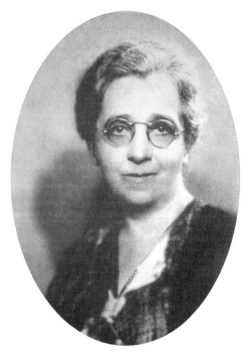

Isabel Maitland Stewart, Sister Domitilla's major instructor, was both mentor and friend. "American nursing's most influential spokeswoman in the area of education for forty-five years," according to historian M. P. Donahue, Isabel Stewart "filled the roles of scholar, author, educator, researcher, administrator, and leader with distinction." She headed Columbia's Department of Nursing Education and developed the first course on the teaching of

Isabel Maitland Stewart, mentor and friend of Sister Domitilla, headed the Department of Nursing Education at Columbia University. (From Donahue MP: Nursing, the Finest Art: An Illustrated History. Second edition. St. Louis: Mosby, 1996, p 343. Copyrighted and used with permission of the author.)

nursing. Sister Domitilla's biographer, Sister Charlotte Dusbabek, asked Stewart to assess her former student's contribution to nursing: "I have always felt that Sister Domitilla had a strong influence in paving the way for other Sisters to get advanced preparation and to join actively in professional associations, where they not only strengthened their own professional competence but contributed much to the work of the group and to nursing generally. Though I am convinced that she was a strong factor in uniting the religious and secular nurse in this country I am not sure I could give you all the reasons for my belief. I know that in many of my travels in Europe and elsewhere, I found a wide gap in such groups, due, I think, to the lack of such leaders."

Shortly after graduating from Columbia in 1920, Sister Domitilla spoke about Columbia's nursing program to religious nursing leaders at a meeting of the Catholic Hospital Association. She listed reasons for them to consider the program, among them, the advantage of interacting with students from a wide array of institutions in America and foreign countries. "Each one had come to get and to give. All had faced the same kind of problems and had come for help in solving them . . . It is a real relief, too, to find that our problems are not peculiar to our own school and we feel encouraged to push on and help solve them for the profession." Sister Domitilla also addressed the lack of cooperation between religious and secular nursing leaders: "On the whole there is not a nice spirit of cooperation and this is detrimental to the progress of nursing. There may be a conflict of judgment and a clash of opinions, but this is to be expected in normal, healthy organizations. This difference of opinion, however, should not foster a spirit of intolerance; it should, on the contrary, make for better progress . . . If we only understood each other a little better, if we only worked together more, great things could be accomplished for human betterment."

Considering all that religious and secular nursing leaders held in common, it might seem inconceivable that they were at odds with each other. They shared a strong commitment of service to suffering humanity and agreed on the need for nursing reform. Nevertheless, these nursing leaders didn't trust each other. Inherent religious and national prejudices were contributing factors. For many Americans with European roots, life experience in the New World had not erased inherited prejudices from the Old World. Moreover, at this time nurses had little contact with persons outside their own institutions. Such narrow perspectives, in the view of nursing leaders, diminished the profession. To promote professional development and build broader relationships, nursing leaders initiated continuing educational opportunities and created professional nursing organizations. These initiatives, enthusiastically endorsed by nurses of all backgrounds, helped bridge differences among members of the profession at a critical time in its history.

The history of nursing in America is closely connected with the Sisters' story of Saint Marys Hospital. Indeed, they grew up together. The pioneer Sisters of Saint Marys were not trained nurses when the hospital opened in 1889. A few weeks of informal instruction from Edith Graham, Rochester's first registered nurse, taught them the rudiments of nursing. Nurses' routine duties included many housekeeping tasks, along with preparing and serving meals. Keeping the patient comfortable, dressing wounds, and giving medications were of foremost importance. Training included such technical skills as using a thermometer, giving enemas, and inserting catheters. Sisters learned nursing skills and procedures on the job from the Doctors Mayo and their physician colleagues. Serving as apprentices to physicians was typical for nurses across the country.

Saint Marys and other hospitals saw a dramatic increase in registrations at that time. Between 1890 and 1910, aseptic technique and other advances created unprecedented medical opportunities. Patients survived surgeries and medical conditions that earlier would have been fatal. The public, no longer in fear of hospitals, sought them out, and institutions multiplied rapidly. The growth of hospitals triggered an increase in nursing schools under owners who quickly recognized the financial advantage of staffing with unpaid student nurses. According to T. E. Christy, in 1890 in the United States and Canada, "there were 35 training schools with 1,552 pupil nurses and by 1900 there were 432 schools with 11,164 students."

At Saint Marys Hospital, where Sisters were the only nurses, Sister Joseph wanted to institute a training school to provide additional staff and give students the special advantage Saint Marys could offer. The Doctors Mayo, however, did not welcome the idea. "Dr. Charlie and I had always done our work with the Sisters' help, and we were much concerned whether anyone could be taught, even by the Sisters themselves, to perform the duties of the nurse as well as they." The Mayos were also concerned about the potential quality of the school in view of the unfavorable reputation held by the rapidly growing nursing schools that operated without established standards or even textbooks. Sister Joseph didn't share the Mayos' doubts about nursing care from laypersons, but she agreed that the lack of teaching standards could pose serious problems. She believed that the quality of the

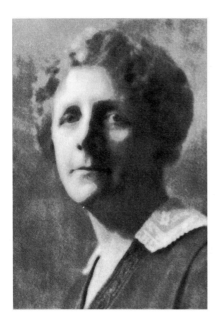

Anna Jamme, first director of Saint Marys School of Nursing, 1906-1912. (From A Century of Caring: 1889-1989. Rochester, MN: Saint Marys Hospital, 1988, p 76.)

school would depend on the kind of person selected to superintend it. In Anna Jamme, a recent graduate of the new Johns Hopkins' Training School for Nurses, she found such a person. In 1906, Anna Jamme became the first director of Saint Marys School of Nursing. Miss Jamme was only on the job for a short period of time before the Mayos and their associates agreed with Sister Joseph. Jamme instituted a 2-year program, including practical experience at the bedside of patients with 142 hours of classroom experience in such subjects as anatomy, bacteriology, physiology, hygiene, practical nursing, and surgical techniques. In her 6 years as superintendent, Anna Jamme saw the school grow, prosper, and take its place as "one of the leaders among institutions of its kind."

Nursing schools without standards or controls proliferated creating serious problems for the fledgling profession. Historians attribute lack of endowments and financial dependence on hospitals as a major problem. The monetary endowments that colleges and universities received from individuals and foundations gave them financial independence. Without endowments, nursing schools were under the control of hospital owners. Many owners, who viewed training schools as business enterprises, had little incentive to change from the profitable apprenticeship system.

Nursing leaders, mostly from major universities, initiated a national movement for nursing reform to address prevailing abuses, such as excessive student hours on duty. The movement gained momentum with the outbreak of World War I, when, "as never before, the country focused attention on issues of public health." Isabel Stewart described the impact of war: "Many of the old barriers of precedent and tradition were broken down and there was a greater willingness to try new methods and to combine forces with others to conserve limited strength and other resources." The war experience brought nursing "into the light of public discussion and criticism. When so many lives hung on the supply of nurses, people were aroused to a new sense of their dependence on the products of nursing schools."

Reformers established committees as vehicles for achieving their goals on state and national levels. Committees documented the current proliferation of training schools, from 1,755 in 1920 to 2,286 in 1927. When the American Nurses' Association surveyed 1,500 training schools in 1925, they found wide variation in entrance requirements and student hours on duty. Educational requirements ranged from completion of 8th grade to earning a high school diploma. The majority required only 1 year of high school. They also found startling differences in student hours of duty, ranging from 25 to 84 hours per week, with an average of 55 hours. "When these figures were compared with the 38-hour week required of most factory workers or with the 42-hour week required of visiting nurses," note historians P. A. and B. J. Kalisch, "one could see why young middle class women were thinking twice about pursuing nursing careers." Standards for educational entrance requirements and student hours on duty became central issues in nursing reform.

Reformers berated hospitals for exploiting student labor but agreed that "one learned how to be a nurse by being a nurse." The value of the experience, they believed, depended on a balance of hours on duty in combination with educational preparation and supervision. Sister Jean Keniry, formerly director of nursing for Saint Marys Hospital from 1978 to 1984, believes she was fortunate to receive a broad education in nursing. She first came to the hospital as a student in the diploma program with its strong emphasis on bedside nursing. Contact with Franciscan Sisters prompted her to enter the congregation, and she went on to earn a baccalaureate and advanced degrees in nursing. Though Sister Jean values the strong academic components of these programs, she hasn't lost an appreciation for lessons learned at the bedside of patients. "Good clinical insight and judgment in a nurse or physician," in her view, "is the ability to reflect and learn from the experience of a wide variety of patients."

When Sister Domitilla returned to Saint Marys from Columbia, she lost little time in implementing what she learned. As instructor of the basic sciences, she introduced laboratory work to the curriculum. "She personally selected the best lecturers from the Mayo Clinic staff and supplemented the lectures with class discussion," an innovation for its time. As the school's director, "Sister Domitilla was particularly interested in faculty development. [Nursing] instructors remembered how she cautioned them about teaching too much: '. . . most young teachers tend to teach more than the student can possibly retain.' Instead, she told them to teach principles and extend the student's interest beyond the last examination. One instructor recalled a favorite message: 'Students aren't sausages to be stuffed and squeezed occasionally. They should be taught so that they can be depended on to continue their learning on their own.'"

Her biographer recorded the impressions of Sister Domitilla's contemporaries: "On a first, casual meeting, Sister Domitilla appeared as a very reserved, non-communicative type of person. Not until one worked with Sister did her strong and pleasing personality become apparent, for she was one who liked to be in the background. The work that she accomplished seemed to be partly hidden by this reserve and by her modesty and humility." Sister Domitilla, aware of her reserve, said of herself, "You know I never talk when I'm working . . . I never talk much when I'm *not* working!" She found it easy, however, to overcome her reserve when she taught or spoke in public. Addressing a group responsible for revising the nursing curriculum, she sensed their apprehension and reminded them about Skippy's prayer in the comic section of the morning paper: "O God, give me strength to brush my teeth every night. But if you can't give me strength to brush my teeth every night, please God, give me strength not to worry about it." She was, as one wag put it, "that near contradiction, a reformer with a sense of humor."

By the early 1930s, Sister Domitilla and many of her peers believed that nursing education was at a new juncture. Isabel Stewart called it a time for action: "If nursing is ever going to justify its name as an applied science," she wrote "some way must be found to submit all our practices as rapidly as possible to the most searching tests which modern science can devise." She urged nurses to take the initiative, not to wait "for someone else outside our own body to recognize our critical situation . . . most of the experimentation that is done will have to be carried on . . . by our own members." Nursing leaders sought advanced degrees in greater numbers. Collegiate nursing programs increased, partly for their academic component and for the opportunities they provided. The Bachelor of Science in Nursing (B.S.N.) was a requisite for admission to graduate school. In contrast, diploma programs, excellent in their own right, didn't fulfill educational requirements for an advanced degree.

"She usually got what she wanted." This comment by a colleague of Sister Domitilla, could apply to her actions prior to becoming Sister Joseph's

successor. She was determined, before
leaving nursing education, to initiate the
Bachelor of Science in Nursing at the
College of Saint Teresa and include clinical
experience at Saint Marys Hospital. She
had only 3 years to achieve her three
objectives: develop a baccalaureate program, initiate it at the college and the
hospital, and secure a director with the
required master's degree. The sequence
of events between 1934 and 1937, in the
middle of the Great Depression, testify
to her ability to get what she wanted.
During the academic year 1934 to 1935,
Sister Domitilla went to Columbia,
earned a Master of Arts degree, and
developed a model for the B.S.N. program.
When she returned, it required all of her
gifts of persuasion and organization to
insert the B.S.N. program at the College

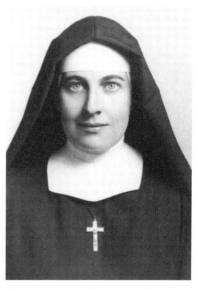

*Sister Ancina Adams, acclaimed
director of the Bachelor of Science in
Nursing (B.S.N.) program at the
College of St. Teresa. (From Saint
Marys Hospital Archives.)*

of Saint Teresa and Saint Marys School of Nursing. She succeeded, and the
new program opened in 1936 under her direction. In the meantime, Sister
Ancina Adams, a gifted instructor in the diploma program, also went to
Columbia and completed the baccalaureate and Master of Arts degrees.
According to plan, in 1937 Sister Domitilla succeeded Sister Joseph and
Sister Ancina became director of the B.S.N. program, a position she held
with distinction for almost 40 years.

Sister Domitilla took immediate responsibility for administering the
hospital. At 81, Sister Joseph appreciated her successor's quiet ability to
effect a smooth transition. At that time Sister Domitilla was one of Mother
Aquinas's elected councilors. The mother superior gave Sister Domitilla
major responsibility for the two and a half million-dollar medical wing
project. Twenty-five years earlier, at a cost of $2.25 million, Sister Joseph
built the surgical pavilion, later named the Joseph Building in her honor.
Acclaimed "the most up to date surgical pavilion in the entire world," the
new building doubled hospital beds to 600. As first assistant to Dr. Will
Mayo, Sister Joseph's personal investment and experience in surgery were
requisites for this achievement. Similarly, Sister Domitilla's personal

investment and years of experience in nursing education and the basic sciences stood her in good stead for building the new medical wing.

Unlike the surgical department, an intrinsic part of Saint Marys from its beginnings, the medical department didn't have a space at the hospital until 1922. Prior to that, Saint Marys was exclusively a surgical hospital because the need for surgical beds left no hospital rooms available for patients with exclusively medical problems. With 300 new beds in the surgical pavilion, the Sisters could expand hospital services. Within the year, renovations provided facilities and patient beds for the medical department whose patients had been housed in several smaller hospitals throughout the city. The medical department welcomed the services Saint Marys offered and the opportunity to have patients in one location.

On the afternoon of the hospital's Golden Anniversary, September 30, 1939, Bishop Francis M. Kelly broke ground for the new medical building. Undoubtedly, some Sisters had misgivings about the project and everyone shared grave concerns about world events beyond the medical center. Only weeks earlier on September 1, 1939, Adolph Hitler ordered German troops to invade Poland; in retaliation, England and France declared war on Germany. The prospect of a second "World War" made it imperative that hospital construction proceed rapidly while building materials were available. Seven months later, Bishop Kelly laid the 1,500-pound cornerstone and spoke about the Sisters' fears and misgivings. "Hesitatingly, the Sisters of Saint Francis launched the project. It was so large that one can readily understand the diffidence superiors might feel in beginning this hospital addition at a time when the future seemed so uncertain. Yet, the need was there; the afflicted required comfort and solace. The love of fellowman was all-important in the reckoning . . . it is this spirit that has built this institution and now bears it on its course."

Physicians from the department of medicine, keenly interested in the medical wing, contacted Sister Domitilla. Several of the specialists spoke to the importance of medical research and requested laboratories for clinical research in the new building. Sister Domitilla welcomed their suggestions and requested permission from the Board of Governors to form a laboratory committee. Though the Board of Governors concurred with their colleagues on the importance of medical research, the outcome of an earlier medical research project at Saint Marys suggested they proceed with caution. In the 1920s, specialists under the leadership of Leonard Rowntree, M.D., created a department of medicine at Saint Marys. Modeled after departments in American universities, it had its own patient care facilities and research laboratories. Mayo medical historian, John L. Graner, M.D., notes that "all of Rowntree's associates came to make noteworthy contributions to the medical knowledge of their day." Unfortunately, the group's real or perceived exclusiveness created conflict within the larger organization and the project ended within a few years. Housing Mayo research facilities in a location outside the Clinic proper would require broad institutional consultation and careful planning.

Sister Domitilla and architects worked with medical specialists to design patient floors and research laboratories in proximity to each other. Such an extensive project, in the opinion of Mayo chief administrator Harry J. Harwick, required a more formal business arrangement with Saint Marys than those of the past. Earlier arrangements, according to Sister Generose Gervais, were quite informal. "The doctors might ask 'for a little space here and there' and the Sisters were happy to provide it whenever they could." Mr. Harwick consulted with the Sisters and made arrangements for the Clinic "to pay a monthly rental of $950 for the thirty-seven regular units of laboratory space and three storage spaces, this rental to include electricity, water, and other general service. It was agreed also that the Clinic would assume responsibility for the maintenance of the laboratories except for that part which properly belongs to the main structure." Significantly, in keeping with their partnership of 52 years, the two institutions sealed the agreement, not with a legal document, but with a handshake. Half a century of partnership hadn't diminished their mutual trust and respect.

Not surprisingly, internal discussions on research laboratories at Saint Marys required considerably more time for the Board of Governors than Mr. Harwick's business arrangements. Indeed, minutes of the Board reflect substantive discussions over a 2-year period. Discussions culminated with the approval of two motions on July 23, 1941. The first motion appointed Charles F. Code, M.D., as "Chairman of the committee directly in charge of the operation of the Mayo Clinic Laboratories, Saint Marys Hospital Division." The second motion, contained in three, single-spaced typed pages, was the carefully crafted plan for governing Saint Marys clinical research operation and an extensive reporting arrangement. In 2004, Hugh R. Butt, M.D., a distinguished Mayo physician since 1934, reflected on the value of the 1941 building: "Mayo laboratories, built for the Francis Building, made an important contribution and served as precursors for future research by clinical specialists. Their legacy lives on in Mayo's remarkable contribution to medical research today."

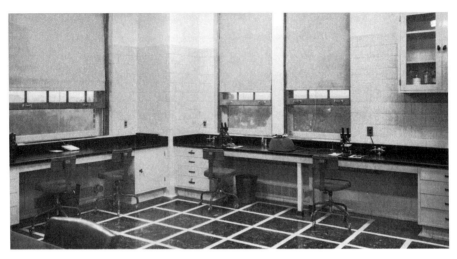

Mayo laboratories, built for the Francis Building, served as precursors for future research by clinical specialists. (From Saint Marys Hospital Archives.)

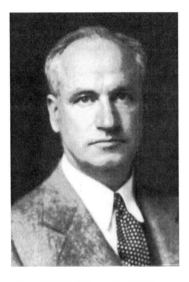

Donald C. Balfour, Sr., M.D., whose distinguished Mayo career spanned 40 years, was a revered colleague of the Franciscan Sisters. (From Nelson CW: Mayo Roots: Profiling the Origins of Mayo Clinic. Rochester, MN: Mayo Historical Unit, Mayo Foundation, 1990, p 133.)

On July 11, 1941, the day before the new wing opened, Sister Domitilla received a gracious note from Donald C. Balfour, M.D. "May I take this opportunity of telling you how much I personally have admired the magnificent way in which you have guided the development of the new wing at Saint Marys Hospital. We are all grateful for the understanding with which you met the innumerable proposals that were made and I know each member of the Staff will make every effort to justify the confidence you have shown in the future of the Clinic and the Foundation by affording us every facility for carrying on our work in the most efficient manner."

Headlines from the *Rochester Post-Bulletin* on July 12, 1941 announced: "New Unit Makes St. Mary's Largest One-Unit Private Hospital in the U.S: Addition Raises Total Capacity to 868 Beds." The article read, "Adding another and significant chapter to the medical history of Rochester, the new addition to St. Mary's hospital stood completed and occupied today, 21 months and 14 days after its construction was launched on the institution's golden anniversary, September 30, 1939."

Press coverage reflected the public's interest, and journalists paid particular attention to the hospital's new clinical features: "Clinical specialties will be segregated in the new addition as follows, first floor, arthritic patients, second, vascular and emergency service, third, gastrointestinal and metabolic disorders . . . the fifth floor is occupied by the obstetrical department, the sixth, pediatric, and the seventh, general. In the tower, adjacent to the floors, were specialized diagnostic and research laboratories." The *Rochester Post-Bulletin* was quite specific: "The third floor, which will be given over to diabetic and gastric cases, has 47 rooms with accommodation for 72 patients. Closely associated with the care of the patients on the third floor are the basal metabolism and blood chemistry laboratories in the tower section. A little kitchenette equipped with stove and refrigerator and a patients' examination room adjoin the laboratories and patient section of the floor. With 46 rooms and accommodations for 69 patients the fourth floor is given over entirely to colon or enterology cases . . . In the tower section, the fourth floor is occupied by laboratories which include rooms for glass blowing, bleeding, hematology, urinalysis, microscope work and gastric research."

The building was indeed a magnificent accomplishment, "So vast," according to the *Rochester Post-Bulletin*, "that it takes literally hours to inspect from top to bottom. The new unit comprises a nine-story tower, and eight-floor west wing, and a nine-floor south wing . . . Architecturally, it conforms with the Renaissance style of the surgical unit, which flanks the tower on the east. On the exterior, the dominating feature of the building is the tower, which rises eight stories from the ground, is eight feet wide and ninety feet deep. Set in a niche at the top of the tower is a statue of Our Lady of Lourdes . . . floodlighted at night. With the completion of the unit, the main entrance for the entire hospital will be shifted to the tower. The [entrance] walk leads to steps of Cold Spring granite, which ascend to an arched bronze doorway of great height. In the clear glass of the doorway are 17 stained glass coats of arms and a central figure of the Sisters' beloved St. Francis. Directly inside the doorway is the vestibule, which is paneled in St. Jeanne marble obtained from Lourdes, France. Cast bronze grilles conceal the radiators and bronze handrails form three lanes leading up a short stairway and into the main lobby. Two stories high and including a balcony, the lobby is finished throughout in marble, American black walnut and ornamental plaster. The floor is of a special Tennessee marble, inset with panels and feature strips of Red and Green Lavento and Verde Antique. Pilasters and columns are all finished in Forest Green with Verde Antique base and Red Lavento bands . . . In the center of the lobby, directly under the balcony, is an information desk, which is of black American walnut."

Opening day of the medical wing, later named the Francis Building in honor of the Sisters of Saint Francis, came and went without a formal dedication, celebration, or public tours. This omission did not occur without comment. The Mayo Board of Governors believed "the public and professional staff should be given an opportunity to view such a magnificent structure and Dr. Balfour and Dr. Henderson were asked to urge the Sisters to have a formal opening to which the public would be invited." Board members had either attended or heard accounts of the surgical pavilion's opening in 1922, when the Sisters sent 2,000 engraved invitations and printed elegant souvenir books for the occasion. All businesses were closed "so that employers and employees might have the time on that day to visit Saint Marys Hospital." During that earlier dedication, 4,000 guests attended the opening and toured the facility. After the public reception, Sister Joseph personally greeted the 500 guests invited to the formal banquet, chaired by Dr. Balfour. Following the memorable presentations, Dr. Balfour told the guests that he had a rather difficult task ahead of him and needed their help. He called on Sister Joseph to speak and with that, the audience rose and applauded until she came from a dark corner of the room. "My very dear friends, I do not deserve the plaudits given to me tonight, but I will take them to distribute them among the Sisters with whom I have worked to make Saint Marys Hospital a house of God and a gateway to heaven for his many suffering children."

The Sisters acknowledged the Board's request and offered informal tours of the new medical building to Mayo staff and their families as well as the public. But the reasons for omitting a formal dedication can only be surmised. Locally, nationally, and internationally, 1941 was a very different time from 1922. World War II raged on a global scale, and the Axis powers of Germany, Italy, and Japan appeared to dominate the struggle. A year earlier, France fell to the Nazis and all of continental Europe was then under Axis powers. England and Russia hung on with help from the United States which formally entered the war 5 months later following Japan's attack on Pearl Harbor, December 7, 1941.

The situation in 1941 was also different for the Franciscan Sisters. They gave thanks for the new medical building and what it would mean for patients and staff. The achievement, however, had been hard won. Six years earlier, in the middle of the Great Depression, the fire marshal publicly condemned the first medical building. The Sisters, already facing bankruptcy, were on notice. The burden of bearing financial responsibility for the congregation and for building a hospital of high quality was a heavy one for Mother Aquinas. Some say she never got over it. While Sister Domitilla and the Saint Marys Sisters probably would have delighted in a

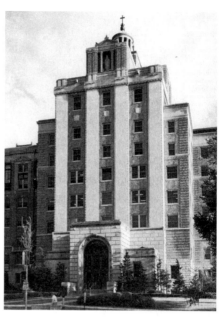

The exterior of the new entrance of Saint Marys Hospital, circa 1941. (From Saint Marys Hospital Archives.)

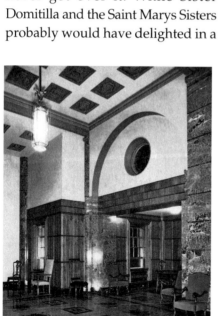

The interior of the new lobby of Saint Marys Hospital, circa 1941. (From Saint Marys Hospital Archives.)

celebration like the one of 1922, it's not surprising that they didn't insist on it.

Instead, the Sisters celebrated the new building informally during those July days. Those who came off night duty cooked their favorite breakfast of fried eggs and had a morning picnic outside at the pergola. Others took time to stroll the tree-lined streets of Rochester, whose population then exceeded 20,000. They walked past the trim lawns and handsome homes of "Pill Hill" and out into the rolling, green countryside. In typical Franciscan fashion, in large and small numbers, the Sisters laughed at stories heard many times before.

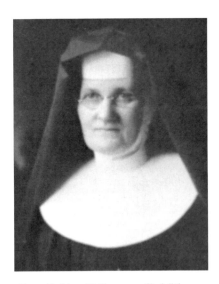

Sister Fabian Halloran, called "the guiding light of patient care," was the last surviving founding Sister of Saint Marys Hospital. (From Whelan E: The Sisters' Story: Saint Marys Hospital—Mayo Clinic 1889-1939. Rochester, MN: Mayo Foundation for Medical Education and Research, 2002, p 100.)

Whenever the Sisters gathered, they shared stories of their beloved Sister Fabian Halloran, last surviving of the founding Sisters, who had died the previous February. This small, gentle woman, called "the guiding light of patient care," was the last hope when things went wrong. Over 50 years a nurse, Sister Fabian's unerring insight into the condition of patients won the complete confidence of nurses and physicians. Her most outstanding trait, however, was kindness. When Sister Fabian retired from nursing, she was appointed superior of the convent. Young Sisters remembered her way of saying, "Child, can I help you?" Sister Antoine Murphy came to Saint Marys in 1938 and remembers Sister Fabian as a "sweet, spiritual woman with swollen feet and hands from arthritis, who met me at the door when I arrived." As a young Sister, Sister Paula Leopold vividly recalls a time that she overslept, "I was scared to death, but what did she say? 'Dear, you must have needed that extra sleep.'"

Sister Domitilla celebrated the new medical wing along with the Sisters and quietly enjoyed listening to the old stories. It was probably the memory of such times together that she recalled in a talk in the summer of 1943. She spoke to a group of Sister teachers who volunteered at the hospital to help ease the critical shortage of employees during World War II: "Remember this is your hospital and while you're here you ought to learn as much about it as you can. Incidentally, you may learn to love it just as much as we do. We have many problems and difficulties all the time, but every once in a while, peace breaks out for no reason at all. In those rare moments, we are terrifically proud of our institution and I hope that you, too, will experience such moments of joy."

ENDNOTES

Page 24   Dusbabek MH: *The Contributions of Sister M. Domitilla DuRocher,
                 O.S.F. to Nursing, 1920-1939.* Unpublished dissertation. Catholic
                 University of America, Washington, DC, 1962, pp 8, 9, 12.

                 Sister Mary Brigh Cassidy, Writings and Speeches, Saint Marys
                 Hospital Archives.

                 Whelan E: *The Sisters' Story: Saint Marys Hospital—Mayo Clinic
                 1889-1939.* Rochester, MN: Mayo Foundation for Medical Education
                 and Research, 2002, pp 124-125.

Page 25   Donahue MP: *Nursing: The Finest Art; An Illustrated History.* Second
                 edition. St. Louis: Mosby, 1996, pp 342-344.

Page 26   Dusbabek (pp 64-65).

Page 27   Christy TE: Nurses in American History: The Fateful Decade, 1890-
                 1900. *American Journal of Nursing* 1975;75:1163-1165.

                 Clapesattle H: *The Doctors Mayo.* Minneapolis: The University of
                 Minnesota Press, 1941, p 499.

Page 28   *A Century of Caring: 1889-1989.* Rochester, MN: Saint Marys Hospital,
                 1988, pp 75-76.

                 *A Souvenir of Saint Mary's Hospital: Founded in Eighteen Hundred
                 and Eighty Nine.* Rochester, MN: Saint Marys Hospital, 1922, pp 29-
                 31.
                 Saint Marys Training School.

                 Kalisch PA, Kalisch BJ: *The Advance of American Nursing.* Third edi-
                 tion. Philadelphia: JB Lippincott, 1995, p 243.

Pages 28-29   Donahue (p 337).

Page 29   Kalisch (pp 243, 254).

                 Interview with Sister Jean Keniry, August 15, 2003.

Pages 29-30   Dusbabek (pp 25, 27).

Page 30   **Whelan E:** *The Sisters' Story: Saint Marys Hospital—Mayo Clinic 1889-1939*, p 127.

                 Dusbabek MH: *The Contributions of Sister M. Domitilla DuRocher, O.S.F. to Nursing*, 1920-1939, p 11.

                 Whelan (pp 126-127).

                 McGinley P: *Saint-Watching.* New York: Viking Press, 1969, p 94.

                 Donahue MP: *Nursing: The Finest Art; An Illustrated History*, pp 419-420.

Page 31   **Johnson V:** *Mayo Clinic: Its Growth and Progress.* Bloomington, MN: Voyageur Press, 1984, p 18.

Page 32   *Saint Marys Alumnae Quarterly* Vol. XXIV, no. 3, July 1940, pp 23-24.

Pages 32-33   **Graner JL:** *A History of the Department of Internal Medicine at the Mayo Clinic.* Rochester, MN: Mayo Foundation for Medical Education and Research, 2002, pp 14-24.

Page 33   Interview with Sister Generose Gervais, July 15, 2004.

                 Mayo Clinic Board of Governors' Meeting Minutes, August 7, 1941.

                 Mayo Clinic Board of Governors' Meeting Minutes, March 1, 1939, July 19, 1939, July 23, 1941, August 7, 1941, and September 17, 1941.

                 Interview with Dr. Hugh Butt, July 14, 2004.

Page 34   **Letter from Dr. Donald C. Balfour to Sister Domitilla DuRocher, July 11, 1941. Saint Marys Hospital Archives.**

Pages 34-35   **New Unit Makes St. Mary's Largest One-Unit Private Hospital in U.S.** *Rochester Post-Bulletin* July 12, 1941, pp 1, 4.

Page 36   **Mayo Clinic Board of Governors' Meeting Minutes, June 1, 1941.**

Pages 36-37   **Saint Marys Hospital Annals, 1922.**

Page 37   **Whelan (p 92).**

"Pill Hill" is the name given the neighborhood around Saint Marys Hospital where many physicians resided.

Page 38   Sister Fabian Halloran, Saint Marys Hospital Archives.

Interview with Sister Antoine Murphy, July 15, 2004.

Interview with Sister Paula Leopold, October 30, 1998.

Talk by Sister Domitilla DuRocher, June 13, 1943. Saint Marys Hospital Archives.

CHAPTER 3

WWII Dedication and Sacrifice

The prospect of fighting another world war divided the nation in the late 1930s. As dictators gained power in Europe and Japan raged through Asia, Americans fiercely debated the merits of intervention versus isolation. Many dismissed President Roosevelt's call for mobilizing at home and aiding allies overseas. The Great Depression sapped the country's confidence, and World War I left Americans wary of involvement. No one was prepared for the kind of attack Hitler unleashed in the summer of 1940. Denmark, Belgium, Holland, Luxembourg, and France collapsed in the face of the Nazi onslaught and British troops on the Continent barely escaped. In the face of such realities, the United States mobilized and extended help to Great Britain.

The United States was transformed by World War II, and so was Saint Marys Hospital. Even the prospect of war influenced every project, major and minor. In Sister Domitilla DuRocher's words, "It was impossible to make a reasonable guess at what the future would bring." The hospital must act with dispatch: first, complete pending projects that improved patient services, next, reorganize the institution for greater efficiency. Such actions, in her view, were the best protection for weathering the uncertainties of war.

Shortly after Sister Joseph Dempsey died, Sister Domitilla called the other Sisters together. She had important things to say and typed her talk in advance. Her remarks went to the heart of their present situation. "When we lost Sister Joseph, we lost the leadership that has made this institution one of the greatest in the world. No matter who is appointed head of the hospital—no one will ever be able to take Sister Joseph's place . . . Yet everyone," she told them, "who is part of the institution wants to maintain its place. There are two ways in which an institution like this can succeed. One is through great leadership—the other is through good organization and administration. It can be done by good organization in which we all pull together. Today we can begin in a small way. We begin today not as a matter of choice but of necessity."

Sister Mary Brigh Cassidy, then faculty member for the school of nursing, was among the Sisters who listened attentively to Sister Domitilla. Years later, after Sister Mary Brigh became hospital superintendent, she would describe her predecessor's challenges. "To her fell the difficult and often unappreciated work of reorganizing a hospital which had grown to a size that made it impossible to function effectively on the informal basis that prevailed through the early years."

Sister Domitilla met these institutional challenges with consummate skill. Interestingly, she had been given the basics of managing a large hospital 20 years earlier as a student in Columbia University's nursing program. At that time, haphazard management prevailed in most hospitals. Mary Adelaide Nutting, founder of Columbia's nursing program, developed a curricular component in hospital administration—the first of its kind. Nurses learned management skills from courses that combined academic principles with hands-on learning at ranking New York hospitals. Sister Domitilla valued the experience. Shortly after graduation in 1920, she spoke to members of the Catholic Hospital Association about Columbia's nursing program. Presciently, perhaps, she called the administrative courses among "the most important in the program."

Sister Domitilla's institutional initiatives brought sweeping changes to the hospital in 1940 and 1941. Major construction went forward with an urgency driven by threatened shortages of materials and labor. While the new medical wing, now the Francis Building, was still under construction, Saint Marys added two operating rooms to the surgical wing. Built in 3 months at a cost of $50,000, the operating rooms had a number of new features, including air conditioning. On another part of the campus, contractors enlarged the power plant and installed a third smokestack. Their next project was the new laundry building. Ruefully, Sister Antoine Murphy remembers her prediction at the time: "Surely, this will be the last large building constructed at Saint Marys."

New organizational structures became a reality as well, among them centralized purchasing, an accounting system, and a personnel department. An advanced telephone system facilitated communication and improved patient services. To head these new departments, Sister Domitilla hired experienced laymen from outside the hospital, an innovation not welcomed in certain quarters.

Some Sisters voiced their concern that such widespread institutional change threatened the spirit of the hospital. Never at a loss, Sister Domitilla called the Sisters together: "We are getting ready to establish a store room and complete our plans for central purchasing and central supplies. Mr. Cox, the accountant who is assisting us, will be here during June and we shall ask him to meet you all and explain the things we are trying to do. It may be of interest for you to know that the plans for the reorganization of accounting and management of supplies, as well as the men we have secured to help us, were approved by Sister Joseph, also by Mother Aquinas [Norton] and Bishop Kelly. So not any of us need to worry about the change in policy. It makes absolutely no difference to us if these men are Methodists, or Jews, or Hottentots. They were not secured to teach religion. They are experts in the things we want done and that is all that matters."

Hiring laypersons as managers of departments, rather than assigning Sisters, undoubtedly received a mixed reaction. This innovation, however, would bear great fruit. As later chapters attest, dedicated lay women and men steadily grew in numbers at the hospital. In the 1960s, for example, when the pool of available Sisters began to ebb, lay colleagues increasingly moved into leadership and staff positions. This partnership of laypersons and Sisters continued to achieve the institution's goal of unstinting service to patients. Today at Saint Marys, able and selfless laypersons carry the mission they inherited from Franciscan Sisters forward into the future.

It is worth noting that the new accounting consultant, Mr. Cox, insisted that the Sisters be compensated for their labors. Prior to this time, they received no remuneration. With this change, Sisters' salaries went directly to the motherhouse and contributed to the needs and works of the congregation, including Saint Marys Hospital.

The hospital's new structures, concrete and organizational, were largely Sister Domitilla's accomplishments. In addition to her considerable abilities, she had a number of factors working in her favor. Almost unlimited authority came with her appointment as superintendent, along with extensive resources to reach her objectives. Importantly, she could expect compliance from every Franciscan. Sisters might disagree with the superintendent's directives, but, by and large, they followed them. Such compliance for strong-minded, decisive women was at times personally difficult. In those years, however, dedication to the institution transcended personal preference. Sister Generose Gervais, who would become hospital administrator in 1971, was among the young Sisters who learned from the example of others. One of her favorite sayings, "Values are caught, not taught," recalls the power of this example.

On the national scene, an event of world proportion settled the nation's debate about going to war. Sunday, December 7, 1941, Japanese forces made a surprise attack on the Naval Base at Pearl Harbor. They sank or damaged 31 ships and demolished 188 aircraft and damaged 159 others. A.E. Cowdrey, M.D., in *Fighting for Life* on military medicine in World War II writes: "Under the ruins or the sea some 2,300 Americans died and 1,100 more were wounded." That same day the Japanese attacked the Philippines, Malaya, Wake Island, Guam, and Hong Kong.

Alberta Rose Krape, 24 years old, joined the Navy in November 1941. She made $70 a month and wore a single gold stripe on her cap, designating her an ensign. (From Life, January 5, 1942, cover photo. Used with permission, Eliot Elisofon/Time & Life Pictures/Getty Images.)

"No American who lived through that Sunday would ever forget it," wrote reporter Marquis Childs. "It seared deeply into the national consciousness, creating in all a permanent memory of where they were when they first heard the news." December 7, 1941, instantly transformed the nation: "It infuriated Americans; it challenged them; it energized them. They began to act as one people, putting the demands of society ahead of their own desires. During the four years following Pearl Harbor, Americans focused their eyes on the war."

As staff from Saint Marys and Mayo Clinic joined the armed forces, employees and Sisters joined to fight for victory on the homefront. Members of a newly established Victory Committee created the first hospital-wide newsletter. *Saint Marys Hospital Bulletin* went to press with two objectives: to keep in touch with nurses and employees in the armed forces and to promote efforts at home for winning the war.

"We are at war," read the first editorial. "Our Government needs everything that's being produced in this country for manufacturing ammunition, guns, and planes. This means life as usual is out of the picture for the duration of the war and increasingly we shall be subjected to lower standards of living and less of everything." The next issue again challenged readers: "There is opportunity for every one of us to make a contribution here in our community to the welfare of the nation at large . . . We must learn the true meaning of sacrifice, of more work, faster work, and of one more job."

Graduate nurses at Saint Marys, like their counterparts across the country, quickly responded to the urgent call for nurses to join the armed forces. When the Japanese attacked Pearl Harbor, the Army nurse corps numbered fewer than 1,000; 6 months later, its rolls soared to 12,000. Seventy-nine thousand nurses served in the armed forces during World War II, often under fire, in field and evacuation hospitals, on hospital trains and hospital ships, and as flight nurses on medical transport planes.

To increase the number of nurses available for both military and civilian service, the government offered free education to nursing students through the Cadet Nurse Corps (CNC). Saint Marys School of Nursing was one of the schools chosen by the government to participate in the program. According to nursing historian Mary Ellen Grobe, the government awarded special recognition to Saint Marys for their curriculum in the specialties in neurology and medicine.

World War II produced heroines among graduates of Saint Marys School of Nursing. Every issue of *Saint Marys Alumni Quarterly* carried new stories of honors, decorations, and adventures. A total of 254 Saint

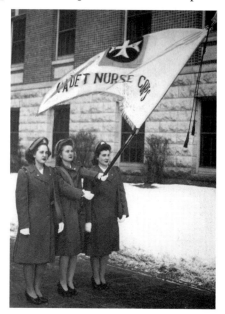

Saint Marys received its first United States Cadet Nurse Corps students in the fall of 1943. (From For 50 Years: Going Forth to Serve. Rochester, MN: Saint Marys School of Nursing.)

Marys alumnae served as nurses in the armed forces. The school's service flag contained one gold star for Jean Tusow, class of 1942, who was killed in a plane crash.

The Saint Marys publications, the *Alumni Quarterly* and *News Bulletin*, literally followed nurses around the globe. Letters from alumnae in the *Quarterly* delighted readers at home and abroad. Lieutenant Mary Grivest wrote from an undisclosed location, "five degrees south of the equator": "The *News Bulletin* and the *Quarterly* arrived several days ago. It is true that we appreciate them much more away from home."

Alumnae read letters of encouragement from graduates not directly engaged in the war. Ellen Ivory Grant wrote from Oakland, California: "I have never lost my deep feeling for Saint Marys and I treasure the happy memories of years spent there . . . So many nurses are called away from home these days. If there are any of the young graduates coming this way, and feel they need a friend, I will be most happy to help them in any way I can. It really doesn't seem so very long ago since I spent some lonesome days in a strange city myself and know that I would have welcomed someone with a kindly interest in my welfare."

Three hundred Mayo physicians were among thousands of doctors who volunteered to serve in the armed forces. Mayo Clinic sponsored three medical units, two in the navy and an army general hospital. Howard K. Gray, M.D., headed a group of eight physicians in Mayo's first navy unit. Sent to Corona, California, and charged with transforming a lavish resort hotel into a navy hospital, they began "without even an aspirin on hand." Mark B. Coventry, M.D., served in the second navy unit, also at Corona, under the command of Waltman Walters, M.D., and wrote about the experience. "There were exactly 18 patients in this massive hotel when we arrived," he recalled. "It was our charge to complete the conversion of this hotel into a functioning naval hospital . . . We saw the naval hospital at Corona grow from the dozen and a half patients to almost 2,000 when we left, a truly phenomenal growth."

Fifteen nurses from Saint Marys served with the Mayo navy units. "It's a wonderful feeling," wrote one new navy nurse, "to see someone you know from the Clinic or Saint Marys." Alumnae wrote home about their experience in Corona: "Nursing is not difficult but very interesting," wrote Frances O'Connor. "Part of our time is spent teaching corpsmen and the patients themselves. Everyone is very cooperative and willing to learn." Ensign Virginia Becker had this to say: "No doubt you would be interested in hearing about our little Mayo Clinic clan out here. I'm enjoying the Navy more everyday. On February 1 we were sworn into the regular Navy Nurse Corps, and that, with Dr. Walters' high approval made me very happy. The vagabond in me is hoping that, among other advantages, this change will make possible either hospital ship duty or overseas duty."

When he heard the news of Pearl Harbor, Charles W. "Chuck" Mayo, M.D., surgeon son of Dr. Charlie, conceived the idea of a Mayo army unit. "The best plan, it seemed to me, was to recruit an entire staff of nurses and doctors at the Clinic and present ourselves as a package to the armed forces." Dr. Chuck and his surgeon colleague, James T. Priestley II, M.D., planned the voluntary unit and invited Saint Marys alumnae to join them. "The Mayo Clinic staff members of this unit wish to extend you an offer to take part in the defense of our country side by side with doctors and nurses whom you know and with whom you have worked."

The Army accepted the generous offer and divided the Mayo General Hospital into two units under the command of Doctors Mayo and Priestley, respectively. Sixty-five Mayo doctors and 75 nurses from Rochester trained for overseas duty, supplemented by other physicians, nurses, and technicians. Both units served in the South Pacific, first in New Guinea and later in the Philippines.

Jermayne Bianchi, class of 1942, was among the Saint Marys nurses who left to join the Mayo unit. "I've waited for this for so long," she told a *Rochester Post-Bulletin* reporter who noted: "Ever since her brother, Captain Willibald Bianchi, was awarded the Congressional Medal of Honor for heroism on Bataan peninsula Ms. Bianchi has been anxious to enter military service . . . Captain Bianchi is a prisoner of war in the Philippines."

Lieutenant Marie Svercl, who served with the Mayo unit, wrote an Easter note in the spring of 1944: ". . . I am on night duty, my second night on and so far everything is quiet. It is a year ago that I was doing my night shift in New Guinea, walking around with a lantern, knee deep in mud and always on the alert for an air raid. How things have changed in that year. They are doing a good job and I hope it continues. I have no idea when I will come home . . . Remember me to the Sisters."

"Today, as in years gone by, the story of American nurses in military service is one of sacrifice, heroism, and signal accomplishments." These words in the *Quarterly* introduced an article about Mary Elizabeth Warren, class of 1942, who received the Silver Star in 1944: Supervisor of an operating room at Saint Marys prior to joining the Army Nurse Corps, she went overseas

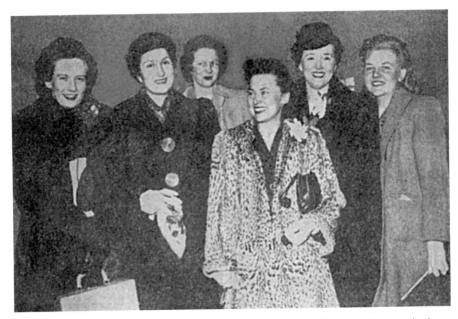

Six Rochester nurses leave for army nurse corps duty at one of the two Mayo units in the South Pacific. (Left to right) Misses Frances Decker, Jermayne Bianchi, Elsie Martinson, Arlene Weston, Ann Sproles, and Gladys Screeden. (From Rochester Post-Bulletin, December 16, 1942. Used with permission.)

almost immediately and was in North Africa until 5 weeks before the invasion of southern France. Her letter of commendation read: "During the period that you were attached for duty in this organization your work was outstanding. Night and day, without thought for yourself you applied your skill for the saving of lives and the prevention of permanent disability, to the utmost possible, in the battle casualties who came under your care."

First Lt. Mary Keily, class of 1930, received the Bronze Star medal in 1944: "Lieutenant Keily distinguished herself as an outstanding officer by the superior performance of her duties as a general duty nurse with the 110th evacuation hospital. Her professional skill, untiring energy and loyal devotion to duty reflect great credit upon herself and the military services." The daughter of John Keily of Rochester, her picture appeared "in a recent issue of the American Journal of Nurses."

That same year, 1944, hundreds of GIs signed a letter in the *Stars and Stripes*, European edition:

"To all Army nurses overseas: We men were not given the choice of working in the battlefield or the home front. We cannot take any credit for being here. We are here because we have to be. You are here because you felt you were needed. So, when an injured man opens his eyes to see one of you . . . concerned with his welfare, he can't but be overcome by the very thought that you are here because it was what you wanted to do . . . [Y]ou endure whatever hardships you must to be where you can do us the most good."

Mayo Clinic and Saint Marys Hospital's contributions to the war effort were not limited to staff members serving in the armed forces. Those who remained in Rochester also served their country with equally dedicated purpose. Dr. Balfour paid tribute to this extraordinary commitment when he spoke to the medical staff at their annual dinner in 1943. "All in all, the participation of the Clinic in this war makes an impressive record. That we have given so much in so many different ways at a time when the registrations are the heaviest in the history of the Clinic is evidence of the strength of our institution in clinical practice, education, and research. The amazing capacity of the staff to carry the extra burden and to work together for a common purpose with a spirit has never been excelled in the history of the Clinic."

For $1.00 a year, Mayo Clinic made an extensive contribution to the government in several areas, among them, top-secret medico-military research. Prior to America's entrance into World War II, Mayo physicians conducted research directly related to the country's preparedness program. Three physicians centered their research on the debilitating effects of high altitude oxygen loss, Walter M. Boothby, M.D., specialist in metabolism and the use of oxygen, W. Randolph Lovelace II, M.D., a resident in surgery and an aviator, and Arthur H. Bulbulian, D.D.S., a specialist in facial prosthetics.

H. Frederick Helmholz, M.D., then in the Department of Physiology, was a neighbor of Dr. Lovelace. "When Randy Lovelace suggested that the physiology of flight would interest me, I started learning about aviation medicine. Randy was enthusiastic and when he got an idea, he wanted to carry it out, and he did." In 1938, the investigators announced the development of an oxygen inhalation mask "which delivered oxygen supplies to aviators at high altitudes." The "BLB Oxygen Mask," widely used by the U.S. Army Air Corps, was named for its designers, Boothby, Lovelace, and Bulbulian.

Jan Stepanek, M.D., a member of Mayo's Section of Aerospace Medicine, notes "the advent of high-performance aircraft in the 1940s with dive-bombing capabilities that taxed the physiological capabilities of the pilots, made research into new strategies for maintaining aviator consciousness a necessity. The Mayo Board of Governors approved the construction of a large human centrifuge capable of simulating the forces encountered by the pilots in flight."

"The first subjects of all aviation medicine experiments were always the physician-researchers; their test-runs were to ascertain that future subjects would not be exposed to undue danger." Both Earl Wood, M.D., the lead investigator in the centrifuge studies, and his associate Edward H. Lambert, M.D., "experienced G-LOC a number of times in their effort to gather data on the physiological effects of G-forces." The human centrifuge was capable a crushing force of 9-G to its occupant, the equivalent of nine times normal body weight. The subject's vital signs, monitored carefully during the exercises, yielded invaluable information for developing the pressurized G-suits for fighter pilots. Nearly unchanged from its original design, the G-suit's basic design "is still in use today in modern fighter aircraft."

The Postanesthesia Recovery Room (PAR) was a striking innovation in surgical patient care. Mayo's chief of anesthesiology, John S. Lundy, M.D., first observed a PAR on a visit to an Army hospital. The centralized ward served all postoperative patients in one location close to the surgical section. Specially trained nurses, equipped to handle emergencies with resuscitative devices, oxygen, and suction equipment, staffed the room. The PAR not only relieved overburdened nursing staffs, but its proximity to surgeons and anesthesiologists saved precious seconds in caring for postoperative patients. Dr. Lundy immediately recommended the arrangement to Saint Marys and the hospital quickly responded. The PAR, instituted on March 17, 1942, "was the first of its kind in civilian hospitals in this country."

In his history of Mayo Clinic, Victor Johnson, M.D., makes this assessment: "Here we have but one of several examples that might be mentioned in which a wartime emergency situation contributed a significant advance in the care of patients and the saving of life, time, and money." Sister Lillian Silver graduated from Saint Marys School of Nursing in 1953 and entered the congregation the same year. First assigned to the PAR, she served in that area for almost 30 years. "We monitored patients' vital signs closely," Sister Lillian recalled. "Anesthesiologists were right around the corner and immediately available when we needed to call on them."

Teaching projects demanded the full-time commitment of a substantial number of Mayo medical personnel. Specialists in medicine and surgery trained some 1,500 officers from the Army, Navy, Public Health Service, and Veterans Administration in courses directly applicable to war conditions. The Mayo program offered courses for up to 6 months in anesthesia, electroencephalography, general surgery and surgical specialties, internal medicine and medical specialties, physical medicine, maxillofacial and plastic surgery, neurologic surgery, roentgenology, surgery of the extremities, and thoracic surgery.

Administrator Harry Harwick was with Mayo during both world wars. "World War I was a difficult time for the Clinic; World War II, unquestionably, was more difficult. As always in wartime, the Clinic contributed heavily in manpower: perhaps a third of our consultants, including ranking members in many specialties; a good third of our Fellows, and, it sometimes seemed, almost every able-bodied man of military age in the non-medical sections. With this depleted staff, we were faced with registrations that reached record numbers . . . Helping to relieve the increasing pressure on our depleted medical staff were certain senior physicians who deferred retirement plans past 65 as their contribution to the war effort and the institution. Some senior physicians, approaching 70, willingly took on workloads more suitable to men half that age, and handled them superbly."

More than 100,000 patients came to Rochester in each of the war years, "about three-hundred per working day. This was more than in any prewar years." With the great reduction in staff members, Clinic physicians carried a tremendous burden. Surgeon O. T. Clagett, M.D. later wrote of that time: "I believe my longest surgical list in one day was 23 major operations. Lists of 15 to 20 operations daily were almost routine. I remember one day I had a list of 19 operations. A visitor in the gallery spoke to me in the course of the day and said, 'I am the medical officer who examined you at Fort Snelling and turned you down as unfit for active military service. I think I made a hell of a mistake.' I can remember times when I had as many as 90 patients on my surgical service at Saint Marys and another 40 at Colonial Hospital at the same time. The postoperative rounds, dressing wounds, administering fluids, writing orders for postoperative care, and all the other details involved a tremendous task for all those involved."

Military needs forced the government to cut civilian goods severely and introduce a rationing system for scarce materials, including food, clothing, and gasoline. Doris Kearns Goodwin describes the rationing system for food and shoes in her book about the homefront in World War II: "In the summer of 1942, the accustomed rhythms of daily life were disrupted in every factory, business, and home by the institution of rationing and price control . . . The first step in developing the rationing system was the creation of a list of essential items in short supply. Each item was then given a price in points, and each man, woman, and child in the country received a book of stamps. The stamps in each ration book—worth 48 points each month, and good for 6 months—could be spent on any combination of goods, from meat, butter, and canned vegetables to sugar and shoes. When a sale was made, the retailer would collect the points and use them to replenish his stocks. Ration books were priceless possessions, as Mrs. Harold Calvert of Oklahoma City found out when her two children ate all the coupons from her first book and she had to present the damaged book before being issued a replacement."

Campaigns for salvaging waste for the war effort were the norm in every home and institution. The first issue of *Saint Marys News Bulletin* announced a new contest, "Saving for Victory." Prizes went for the best suggestions on "saving waste, economical practices, and substitutes for materials in short supply." The Victory Committee incorporated employees' suggestions in an exhibit for the American Hospital Association's annual meeting. They received high praise. "The 'War on Waste' exhibit of Saint Marys Hospital, Rochester, Minnesota graphically demonstrates ways to

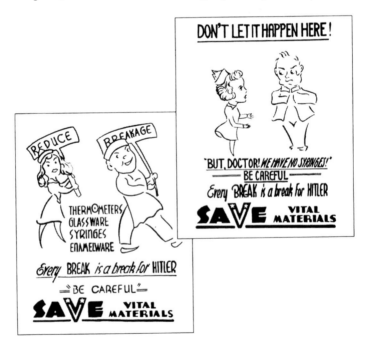

Posters throughout Saint Marys Hospital reminded staff that conservation was essential to victory. (From A Century of Caring: 1889-1989. Rochester, MN: Saint Marys Hospital, 1988, p 58.)

save hospital money and materials. A visit to this exhibit will be well worth the cost of coming to St. Louis."

Mayo's four-page brochure, "Our War Time Conservation Program," also contained many employee suggestions. "Clean out your desk and stationery cupboard," they urged readers, "remove all unnecessary and excess supplies, and return them to the stock room. Return pencil stubs to the stock room. Holders will be supplied and the pencils used in certain sections . . . Pick up from the floor paperclips and rubber bands. They are now priceless because we cannot buy them anymore . . . Cotton may be inserted in the ends of the fingers of rubber gloves to prevent injury to the gloves by sharp fingernails."

Early in the war, Sister Domitilla and Sister Antonia Rostomily, director of Saint Marys School of Nursing, discussed how they might assist Japanese American nursing students on the West Coast. The students were among 120,000 persons of Japanese descent removed from their homes, jobs, and schools by military order to live in "relocation camps." In response, civic, religious, and academic leaders formed the National Japanese American Student Relocation Committee (NJASRC) to help American-born children of Japanese immigrants relocate in colleges and universities. "Nursing schools were perhaps the most reluctant to accept Japanese-American young women," wrote NJASRC member John Province. "Many such schools were fearful of the reaction of patients if these girls were assigned to care for them."

Saint Marys Hospital's experience with international patients made it a desirable setting and the

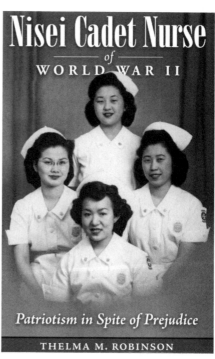

Nisei Cadet Nurses in student uniform, Saint Marys School of Nursing, 1945. Top: Mary (Izumi) Tamura. Middle, left to right: Mary (Sagata) Tamura, Ida (Sakohira) Kawaguchi. Bottom: Sharon (Tanagi) Aburano. (From Robinson TM: Nisei Cadet Nurse of World War II: Patriotism in Spite of Prejudice. Boulder, CO: Black Swan Mill Press, cover photo. Used with permission.)

hospital received approval from the Army and Navy. "Immediately," wrote Sister Antonia, "many requests of students at the relocation site were received." Fifteen of them, "carefully selected for their scholastic ability, educational, and social background" were accepted. In addition, Saint Marys hired seven Japanese-Americans for several positions: nursing instructor, night supervisor, a dietitian, three head nurses, and a secretary for the School of Nursing. Sister Antonia praised all of these women: "We have found them to be loyal, ambitious, outstanding in their scholastic accomplishments as well as skillful in their nursing care of patients. Patients, students, and instructors have paid them many tributes. They should certainly be commended for their splendid adjustment during this trying period of war."

The arrangement with Japanese-American nurses was a mutually beneficial one. "The hospital was desperate for nurses," recalls Sister Amadeus Klein, "Sisters were almost the only graduate nurses on the floors and did literally everything—they cared for patients, made the beds, gave the baths, sterilized instruments, took patients to surgery, picked up medications, and looked after their own supplies."

When the fourth floor of the new medical wing opened, the hospital's capacity grew to 820, an increase of 102 patient beds (Table 1). Even then,

Table 1. A Chart From Saint Marys Annals of 1943

	1941-1942	1942-1943
Daily average patients	618	786.9
Total bed capacity	718	820
Total cribs	49	56
Private duty staff	204	131
Head nurses	32	37
Assistant head nurses	26	14
Instructors	6	9
Supervisors	9	12
General duty nurses	66	7
Student nurses	261	334
Aides	25	56
Desk clerks	8	10
Orderlies	7	3

patient demands exceeded rooms available and required extra beds in the halls. A significant factor in soaring patient numbers at Saint Marys and hospitals across the country was the introduction of prepaid hospitalization.

The Blue Cross plan for prepaid hospitalization had its roots in the late 1930s, the end of the Great Depression. Financial problems of the Depression made it impossible for many families to afford medical care—sometimes with devastating consequences. As the economy recovered and jobs and wages increased, Americans began to invest in prepaid hospitalization. Writing for *Hospital Progress*, John O'Brien described the growth of Blue Cross: "Between January 1, 1937 and January 1, 1942, eight million people subscribed to this voluntary method of pre-paid hospitalization. From humble beginnings it outlined an entirely new principle in paying for needed hospitalization and blazoned its way across the sky in the name of Blue Cross. The Blue Cross now protects 9 million members, one million new members secured this benefit in the past ninety days."

Sister Antoine was head nurse on Second Medical, a vascular floor with responsibility for all medical emergencies. "Intensive Care Units [ICUs] were not yet available for acutely ill patients and private duty nurses were in short supply. Caring for our patients was a serious problem and, as the saying goes, 'necessity is the mother of invention.'" Sister Antoine piloted a new model for patient care called "nursing teams" on one of the hospital wings she supervised. Each team served a designated group of patients. Nurses with different levels of preparation worked together: a graduate nurse headed the team assisted by student nurses, aides, and orderlies. The new model significantly improved patient care and Sister Antoine was soon asked to speak about the pilot program at a district meeting of the Minnesota Nursing Association.

As a member of the congregation's leadership group, Sister Domitilla had regular contact with Mother Aquinas. She persuaded her to ask Sisters who were teachers to volunteer at Saint

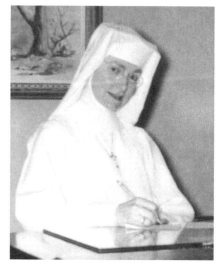

Sister Antoine Murphy was head nurse on the vascular floor, with responsibility for all medical emergencies. (From Saint Marys Hospital Archives.)

Marys during the summer. In the spring of 1943, Mother Aquinas wrote to the Sisters: "It is necessary that some of our teaching Sisters help take care of patients at Saint Marys Hospital during the summer. Will any Sister willing to do this, please let me know at once." Forty Sisters volunteered; twenty-nine served as nurse's aides on the floors, while the others worked in the business office, dietary department, and sewing room.

Sister Domitilla gave the volunteers Sunday morning conferences entitled, "A Bird's Eye View of the Hospital." Her first objective was to clarify the hospital's relationship to Mayo Clinic: "Sometimes we hear Sisters say if it weren't for the Sisters there would be no Mayo Clinic. We really can not make that assumption. The Mayos were leaders. If they had not the Sisters of Saint Francis to pull with them, they would have found someone else and we should be humble enough to recognize that fact. We should also be eternally grateful for the circumstances which enabled us to pull together . . . we have second place in a great medical center recognized all over the world. By that I mean, when a patient comes to Rochester, he comes because of the Mayo Clinic, not because of Saint Marys Hospital."

Sisters Audrey Zenner and Climacus Hund, who volunteered for succeeding summers, found the experience helpful in their classrooms. Delayed by school commitments, Sister Jacqueline Farrell was disappointed she missed nurse's aide training, but gained in her understanding of the hospital from work in central supply. Like other nurse's aides, Sister Margaret Louise Branton was anxious when she began on the floors: "I was nervous the first time I was called to a patient's room. I expected the worst. Imagine my relief when the patient asked, 'Sister, would you please close the window?'"

Sisters Mary Beth Modde and Johnita Klingler also had anxieties about their assignment. Bookkeeping teachers, they were assigned to work all night in the cashier's office on the hospital's books. Their location near the open doors of the main entrance was a concern. Sister Mary Beth recalled one night on duty: "It was about one in the morning and Sister Domitilla came to see how we were getting along. We told her we were worried about the cashiers' window being open at the bottom. She said, 'Oh, you really don't need to worry about that—the glass is completely bulletproof.' Neither of us found the information particularly reassuring."

Sister Amadeus, who loved teaching at St. John's grade school in Rochester, had no thought of becoming a nurse when she volunteered for the summers. Along with two other summer volunteers, Sisters Florence Zweber and Cecile Ewald, the experience inspired her to become a nurse.

All three women, as future chapters will attest, made significant contributions to Saint Marys in their new role.

Sister Michaea Byron did not leave teaching, but her volunteer experience changed her life in other ways. "The summers at Saint Marys were an opportunity to renew gratitude for good health, so often taken for granted, and the chance to know many of our Sister nurses. It made me feel such a part of Saint Marys Hospital—and that continues to this day." Some 40 years later, this college professor became a long-standing member of the Saint Marys Hospital Sponsorship Board and subsequently served as coordinator of health ministry for the diocese of St. Cloud, Minnesota.

Sister Mary Carol Kelly had always wanted to be a nurse, but Mother Aquinas assigned her to teach. She volunteered at Saint Marys to decide if she wanted to request a nursing assignment. "The Saint Marys volunteer experience taught me an important lesson. Nursing was not my calling. I liked teaching and, besides, those hospital Sisters never had any time off." Nevertheless, she delighted in telling stories like this one of her hospital experiences:

"One day a lovely woman came out of her husband's hospital room looking very disturbed. I asked if I could help. She was upset about her husband's health and his behavior. He was an Irishman, O'Shaunessy by name. Mr. O'Shaunessy was ill with yellow jaundice and very angry

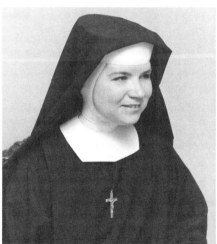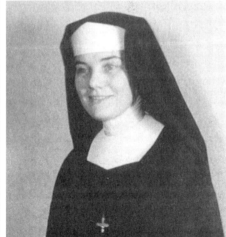

Sisters Michaea Byron (left) and Mary Carol Kelly (right) were among many teaching Sisters who volunteered at Saint Marys Hospital during the summers. (Courtesy of Sister Mary Carol Kelly and Sister Michaea Byron.)

about his condition. In fact, his wife told me, he swore at every person who entered his room and begged me not to see him. I told her not to worry and walked right into the room: 'Mr. O'Shaunessy,' I said, 'I understand you have a new system of cussing, can I hear it? I'm not sure just how Mr. O'Shaunessy recovered from his illness, but I'm sure he was cured of cussing—at least at Saint Marys."

Like Sister teachers, almost every American enlisted as a volunteer during the war. It was the rare person, man, woman, or child, who was not a volunteer at some time. Hospitals were particularly grateful to the American Red Cross for recruiting and training volunteers. Early in 1940, aware of the nursing shortage, the Red Cross designed a volunteer nurse's aides course. Dedicated women of all ages and backgrounds responded with enthusiasm. Saint Marys had a full array of volunteers: nurse's aides, Girl Scouts, and Grey Ladies. Lauretta Schmitt served as instructor and volunteer coordinator. These volunteers, though numbering fewer than 200, contributed thousands of service hours and significantly eased the nursing shortage at Saint Marys.

Lauretta Schmitt introduced volunteer nurse's aides to employees through the *News Bulletin*: "'Have you wondered who the ladies are in the pretty blue pinafores and white blouses?' They come to Saint Marys as part of the nation-wide program sponsored by the American Red Cross to alleviate the acute nursing shortage. Highly dedicated, many of them work much longer than their assigned hours. Probably news to most readers, many nurse's aides from other cities, when in Rochester, call the Red Cross to volunteer at Saint Marys. 'The next time you pass by one of the Volunteer Nurse's Aides or see one in line in the cafeteria, how about a kindly word of encouragement, a word of help to let them know we appreciate their assistance and presence?'"

The first Rochester class of Grey Ladies, 27 in all, graduated in June 1945. Like the nurse's aides, they directly assisted patients. Grey Ladies accompanied patients to the Clinic and x-ray department, to boarding houses and trains. They also fed incapacitated adults and children, wrote letters, read to patients, and cared for their flowers. As one head nurse gratefully remarked, "Grey Ladies are tremendous help to an overburdened nurse."

Girl Scouts were also eager to serve. High school Scouts initiated the idea of a hospital volunteer program at Saint Marys. After an introductory course from Sister Mary Brigh, Scouts served on the wards, in the pharmacy, and in central supply. Called "Pinafore Girls" for their uniforms, the Scouts worked after school and weekend mornings.

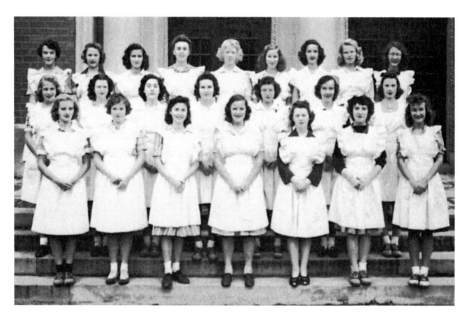

Pinafore Girls, teenagers from the Rochester area, helped the hospital run efficiently during World War II. (From A Century of Caring: 1889-1989. Rochester, MN: Saint Marys Hospital, 1988, p 58.)

Barbara Berkman Withers, grandniece of Dr. Will Mayo, volunteered in pediatrics. Many years later, when asked about her experience, she exclaimed, "I'll never forget it! It was my first experience in a hospital. I worked in Peds and never dreamed children could be so ill. I felt great empathy for them." The experience made a lasting impact on this Rochester resident who has made volunteerism a lifelong commitment.

Girl Scout Jean Rynearson Michaels, like her friend "Barbie" Withers, also made community service a lifelong commitment. Jean recalled working in the central service department with Sister Bertilla Lebens, a stern taskmaster. She accompanied doctors on patient rounds with the instrument cart. One of her jobs was to count every instrument used on a patient. "I thought I was counting instruments to make sure they weren't left inside the patient, but one of the doctors informed me, I was counting them for billing purposes!"

A highlight of her experience happened one day as she did routine work in central service. Doctors and nurses excitedly crowded into the room—they called her over "to witness an historic event." The first units of penicillin arrived on April 28, 1944.

Penicillin, like the PAR, was one of several dramatic medical advances developed during World War II. A British discovery, it could be produced only in miniscule quantities in 1942. The United States government initiated the Committee on Medical Research (CMR), which brought the production of penicillin to a large scale. Penicillin treatment of military casualties began in April 1943. The treatment allowed evacuation of wounded men from military zones to the United States by air with little danger of major wound infection. Saint Marys was one of the first civilian hospitals to receive the drug, but a few months later it went to almost 3,000 hospitals. By the end of the war, penicillin was an acknowledged success and available to the entire population.

Organized national research was successful in developing other drugs during World War II, such as the sulfa compounds. Because of the new sulfa compounds, not a single limb was lost from posttrauma infections at Pearl Harbor. Quinine for the treatment of malaria in the South Pacific was another important advancement. In 1944, Mayo physicians Corwin Hinshaw, M.D., and William Feldman, M.D., gave the "first therapeutic application of streptomycin to treat tuberculosis." The patient, a 21-year-old woman in the last stages of pulmonary tuberculosis, was cured. "Until then, the scientific community was convinced that nothing would ever kill tubercle bacilli in humans."

World War II transformed Saint Marys Hospital. Medical advances such as penicillin, sulfonamide, and other "miracle drugs," revolutionized patient care. Psychiatry and physical medicine, which emerged from the war as new medical specialties, became important components of patient services at the hospital. Unprecedented patient numbers during the war and an acute shortage of nurses prompted new models of patient care, among them, the postanesthesia recovery room, a precursor of the intensive care unit. The volunteer movement in health care also had its origins in World War II. A wide variety of women, including Franciscan Sisters, volunteered as nurse's aides and served in other capacities. These medical advances and innovations became permanent fixtures in health care and signaled greater innovations for the future.

Just as many Americans could recall where they were when they learned of the attack on Pearl Harbor, December 7, 1941, the same could be said of V-J Day, August 14, 1945, when Japan announced unconditional surrender. The war was over and the celebrations began. Sister Antoine remembers going to special services in the Saint Marys Chapel. "The organist was playing a rousing hymn of jubilation when the stop went out. The noise was deafening and lasted a long time—and everyone smiled through it all."

After the celebrations, most Americans only wanted to put the war behind them and go forward with their lives. At the same time, many pondered the meaning of the experience. Perhaps such thoughts prompted a reflection from pediatrician Benjamin Spock, M.D., who joined Mayo's Department of Psychiatry after his discharge from the Navy. "I think, as in most wars, mental health for the majority of Americans improved. During wartime there is less suicide, less crime. People were friendlier; they took care of each other. It's a horrid thing to realize that during wartime people are mentally more healthy than they are during peacetime, especially in a country where so many people live relatively comfortable lives. This kept making me come back to the conclusion that our species is designed to cope with adversity rather than take it easy."

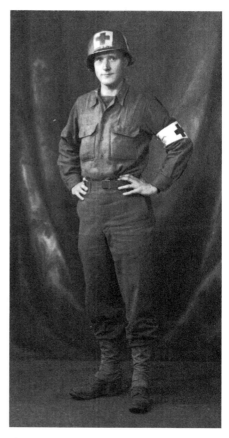

In the summer of 1945, William M. McConahey, M.D., then a physician with the occupation forces in Germany, wrote a memoir of his experiences as a battalion surgeon. He landed in France on D-Day Plus Two, served the casualties of war through Normandy and the Battle of the Bulge, and witnessed the liberated concentration camp at Flossenberg. After the war, Dr. McConahey joined Mayo in Internal Medicine and Endocrinology and his memoirs, entitled *Battalion Surgeon*, were published in 1966. Acclaimed by readers, as "the best of its kind," one wrote, "You have captured the horror and tragedy and heroism and suffering of war." Dr. McConahey later spoke of the experience: "They

Captain William McConahey, M.D., serving in France, September 25, 1944. (Courtesy of Peter M. McConahey.)

call you a battalion surgeon," he said, in his self-deprecating way, "I didn't know surgery; really, I was simply trying to save lives."

Attempts to put the war in perspective began before hostilities ended. Lieutenant Shirley Newton was with the Army Nurse Corps in Iran in 1944 when she wrote to the *Quarterly*:

"I like it here, but the good old U.S.A. is a most wonderful place. I think we were born and raised in heaven and just didn't know it . . . Give my regards to everyone."

ENDNOTES

Page 43   Schneider CJ, Schneider D: *World War II: An Eyewitness History.* New York: Facts on File, Inc., 2003, p 63.

Pages 43-44   Sister Domitilla DuRocher Papers. Saint Marys Hospital Archives.

Page 44   Sister Mary Brigh Cassidy Papers. Saint Marys Hospital Archives.

Kalisch PA, Kalisch BJ: *The Advance of American Nursing.* Third edition. Philadelphia: JB Lippincott, 1995, p 210.
"The editor of the *Modern Hospital* deplored the presence of 'disreputable hospitals' in a stinging 1914 editorial. 'There are many hospitals in this country that are a disgrace to everyone connected with them. Some are immoral in one way, some in another, and some in their very essence and in every way.'"

Stevens R: *In Sickness and in Wealth: American Hospitals in the Twentieth Century.* New York: Basic Books, 1989, p 74.
"The wide variety of backgrounds of hospital superintendents and the enormous range of institutions made it difficult to say there was one general administrative role. Over half the superintendents who belonged to AHA in 1916 were graduate nurses. The first hospital administration and nursing-school administration teaching program . . . was established (for nurses) at Columbia Teachers College in 1900 . . . Interestingly, present-day hospital administration textbooks do not mention this program in presenting the history of management education. Nursing administration has indeed rarely been viewed as fully as 'administration,' for reasons which go far beyond the role itself and include strong elements of gender prejudice."

New Operating Rooms Opened at St. Mary's. *Saint Marys Alumnae Quarterly* Vol. XXIV, no. 4, October 1940, pp 14-15.

Interview with Sister Antoine Murphy, February 18, 2004.

Page 45   Sister Domitilla DuRocher Papers. Saint Marys Hospital Archives. May 12, 1939, presentation.

Interview with Sister Generose Gervais, July 15, 2004.

Page 46   Cowdrey AE: *Fighting for Life: American Military Medicine in World War II.* New York: Free Press, 1994, p 31.

Goodwin DK: *No Ordinary Time*. New York: Touchstone Books, 1995, p 290.
Marquis Childs' quote.

Schneider CJ, Schneider D: *World War II: An Eyewitness History*, p 185.
American response to Pearl Harbor.

Pages 46-47   *Saint Marys Hospital Bulletin* Vol. I, no. 1, May 1942, p 3.

Page 47   Schneider and Schneider (p 142).
Army nurses.

Grobe ME: *Development of Nursing at Mayo Clinic* [videorecording]. Rochester, MN: Mayo Foundation for Medical Education and Research, 1993.

Pages 47-48   *For 50 Years: Going Forth to Serve*. Saint Marys Hospital Archives.
Saint Marys School of Nursing publication celebrating their Golden Anniversary, 1956.

Page 48   Lt. Mary Grivest, July 22, 1944. *Saint Marys Alumnae Quarterly* Vol. XXVIII, no. 3, October 1944, p 13.

Ellen Ivory Grant. *Saint Marys Alumnae Quarterly* Vol. XXVI, no. 2, April 1942, pp 12-13.

Reminiscences of Mark B. Coventry, M.D., May, 1970. Reminiscences of Edward N. Cook, M.D., December, 1970. Mayo Historical Suite.
Mayo Naval Medical Units in World War II.

Pages 48-49   F. O'Connor, N.N.C.U.S., Ensign Virginia Beck, U.S.N. *Saint Marys Alumnae Quarterly* Vol. XXVI, no. 4, October 1942, p 14.

Page 49   Mayo CW: *Mayo: The Story of My Family and My Career*. Garden City, NY: Doubleday, 1968, pp 1-2.

Saint Marys Alumnae Quarterly Vol. XXVI, no. 1, January 1942, p 3.
Nurses' invitation to join Mayo Unit.

Nelson CW: *Mayo Roots: Profiling the Origins of Mayo Clinic*. Rochester, MN: Mayo Historical Unit, Mayo Foundation, 1990, pp 128-129.
Mayo units in the Pacific.

Rochester Post-Bulletin December 16, 1942. **Mayo Historical Suite.** Jermayne Bianchi.

Lt. Marie Svercl, March 11, 1944. *Saint Marys Alumnae Quarterly* **Vol. XXVIII, no. 2, April 1944, p 14.**

Pages 49-50   *Saint Marys Alumnae Quarterly* **Vol. XXVIII, no. 4, October 1944, pp 18-19.**
Mary Elizabeth Warren's award noted.

Page 50   *Rochester Post-Bulletin* **September 27, 1945. Saint Marys Hospital Archives.**
Mary Keily's award noted.

Pages 50-51   *Stars and Stripes*, **European edition, October 21, 1944. Quoted in Schneider CJ, Schneider D:** *World War II: An Eyewitness History*, **p 175.**

Page 51   **Balfour Papers. Mayo Historical Suite.**

World War II Papers. Mayo Historical Suite.

Interview with H. Frederick Helmholz, M.D., August 23, 2005.

Pages 51-52   **Stepanek J: Aviation Medicine at Mayo.** *Minnesota Medicine* **2003 Sept; 86:44-46.**

Page 52   *Reaching New Heights: Secret Stories of the Mayo Clinic Aero Medical Unit* [videorecording]. **Rochester, MN: Mayo Foundation for Medical Education and Research, July 15, 2002.**

Nelson CW: *Mayo Roots: Profiling the Origins of Mayo Clinic*, **pp 322-325.**

A Century of Caring: 1889-1989. **Rochester, MN: Saint Marys Hospital, 1988, p 62.**

Johnson V: *Mayo Clinic: Its Growth and Progress.* **Bloomington, MN: Voyageur Press, 1984, pp 32-33.**

Interview with Sister Lillian Silvers, August 30, 2006.

Pages 52-53   *Mayo Foundation War News Letter* **February 1944, pp 1-3, 6, 7.**

Page 53   Harwick HJ: *Forty-Four Years With the Mayo Clinic: 1908-1952.*
                   Rochester, MN: Whiting Press, 1957, p 33.

                   Johnson V: *Mayo Clinic: Its Growth and Progress.* Bloomington, MN:
                   Voyageur Press, 1984, p 37.
                   On Dr. Clagett.

Pages 53-54   Goodwin DK: *No Ordinary Time*, p 356.

Page 54   Saint Marys Hospital Annals, 1942.
                   On to Victory Committee established at Saint Marys Hospital, January
                   19, 1942.

                   The Forty-fourth Annual Convention of the American Hospital
                   Association. *Bulletin of the American Hospital Association* October
                   12, 1942. Saint Marys Hospital Archives.

Page 55   Our War Time Conservation Program. World War II Papers. Mayo
                   Historical Suite.

                   American-Japanese Students. Saint Marys Hospital Annals, 1943.

                   Provinse JH: Relocation of American College Students: Acceptance
                   of a Change. *Higher Education* 1945 Apr 16; 1 no. 8:1-4.

Pages 55-56   *Saint Marys Alumnae Quarterly* Vol. XXVIII, no. 2, April 1944, p 4.

Page 56   Changes in the Nursing School Faculty. Saint Marys Annals, 1944.

                   Interview with Sister Amadeus Klein, January 22, 2004.

                   Saint Marys Hospital Annals, 1943.
                   Saint Marys Hospital Statistics for 1941-1942, 1942-1943.

Page 57   O'Brien J: The Blue Cross Plans. *Hospital Progress* 1942 Apr; 23 no.
                   4: 116.
                   Phenomenal growth of health plans.

                   Interview with Sister Antoine Murphy, January 21, 2004.

Pages 57-58   March 28, 1943 letter of Mother Aquinas Norton. Archives of the
                   Sisters of Saint Francis, Assisi Heights, Rochester, Minnesota.

Page 58   **A Bird's Eye View of Saint Marys Hospital, June 13, 1944. Sister Domitilla DuRocher Papers, Saint Marys Hospital Archives.**

Interview with Sister Climacus Hund, January 21, 2004.

Interview with Sister Audrey Zenner, January 19, 2004.

Interview with Sister Jacqueline Farrell, January 28, 2004.

Interview with Sister Margaret Louise Branton, January 18, 2004.

Interview with Sister Mary Beth Modde, January 28, 2004.

Interview with Sister Amadeus Klein, January 22, 2004.

Page 59   Interview with Sister Michaea Byron, November 15, 2004.

Pages 59-60   Interview with Sister Mary Carol Kelly, January 19, 2004.

Page 60   **Schmidt LM: The Volunteer Nurse's Aides.** *Saint Marys Hospital News Bulletin* **January 1943, p 7.**
Nurse's aides.

American Red Cross Volunteer Nurses Aides. *Olmsted County Chapter* **1945 Feb;1 no. 1:1-2.**

Annual Report of Red Cross Volunteers Nurse's Aides and Grey Ladies. Saint Marys Hospital Annals, 1945.

Pages 60-61   Interview with Barbara Berkman Withers, November 11, 2004.

Page 61   Interview with Jean Rynerson Michaels, November 18, 2004.

Annual Report of the Girl Scout Volunteers Service at Saint Marys Hospital. Saint Marys Hospital Annals, 1944.

Pages 61-62   **Cowdrey AE:** *Fighting for Life: American Military Medicine in World War II,* **pp 187-188.**

Page 62   **Stevens R:** *In Sickness and in Wealth: American Hospitals in the Twentieth Century,* **pp 201-202.**

Key Dates for Mayo Clinic. 2. Mayo Historical Suite.
Streptomycin.

Important Dates 1944. **Saint Marys Hospital Annals, Saint Marys Hospital Archives.**

Interview with Sister Antoine Murphy, October 16, 2004.

Page 63   Benjamin Spock. In Hoopes R: *Americans Remember the Home Front: An Oral Narrative.* New York: Hawthorne Books, 1977, p 178. Quoted in Schneider and Schneider: *World War II: An Eyewitness History,* p 92.

Martin MJ: A *View of the First 50 Years of Psychiatry and Psychology at the Mayo Clinic.* Rochester, MN: Mayo Foundation for Medical Education and Research, 1997, p 12.

Pages 63-64   McConahey WM: *Battalion Surgeon.* Privately published in Rochester, MN, 1966.

Dr. William M. McConahey: *Experiencing War: Stories from the Veterans History Project* (Library of Congress), p 1. Available from: http://lcweb2.loc.gov/cocoon/vhp-stories/loc.natlib.afc2001001.01026/

Page 64   Lt. Shirley A. Newton, A.N.C., June 6, 1944. *Saint Marys Alumnae Quarterly* Vol. XXVII, no. 3, July 1944, p 17.

CHAPTER 4

Unlikely Agents of Change

*W*orld War II transformed the United States. Americans subordinated private lives to serve a public duty and found themselves capable of meeting enormous challenges. Military assignments introduced them to new people and unknown places in their own country and around the world. The experience changed citizens' perceptions of themselves, as well as of America and its potential. Postwar opportunities abounded in education and employment, and Americans seized them with new confidence. Postwar optimism, however, was largely limited to the United States. For most of the world, the end of the war was fraught with uncertainty and tension. Indeed, many of today's worldwide social and political problems have their roots in World War II.

Overall, 50 million people died and millions more were displaced by World War II. In the wake of this turmoil, Communism spread across the globe. Concurrently, the colonial empires of Britain, France, and Holland crumbled, and overseas possessions of other European nations agitated for independence. A Cold War between the United States and the Soviet Union threatened worldwide nuclear disaster for over 30 years. The demise of Communism in Eastern Europe ultimately ended the Cold War, but not global instability. Smaller states threatened nuclear reprisal and international terrorism became and remains a growing menace.

In striking contrast, science and technology created a world of their own. Historians J. Bordley and A. M. Harvey describe this phenomenon: "Through these years of turmoil and threats of a nuclear war, science and technology advanced at a pace never before imagined and with autonomy oblivious to the stresses of the sociopolitical environment." Medical science moved forward with new momentum: "The secrets of genetics were unraveled; . . . new viruses were brought to light; new protective vaccines were developed . . . artificial kidneys, heart-lung machines, and cardiac pacemakers were devised; the heart could be opened for repair." Hospitals expanded services and technology and "became the center of practice for proliferating numbers of specialists; and all types of physicians and surgeons were dependent upon the facilities and services of a hospital for the care of their seriously ill patients."

Saint Marys Hospital was in a good position to incorporate new medical advances. The 1941 medical wing, planned in collaboration with Mayo physicians, anticipated postwar needs. Upon learning of a proposed medical wing, Mayo specialists initiated meetings with Sister Domitilla. To facilitate clinical research, they recommended placing medical laboratories in close proximity to specialized patient floors. Sister Domitilla concurred with their recommendation, as did the Mayo Board of Governors, and the design went forward.

The Sisters continued to provide state of the art surgical facilities. In 1940, Saint Marys added two operating rooms with an important new feature—air conditioning. Saint Marys was the first hospital in the United States to establish a postanesthesia recovery room (PAR). The PAR served all postoperative patients in one location, close to the surgical section. By 1947, the surgical suite had three more operating rooms, two for urology and one for cystoscopy.

Surgery was not alone in advancing the art of medicine. As early as 1922, Sister Joseph asked for a psychiatric unit in the new surgical building, later the Joseph Building. At that time, mentally ill patients went to State Hospitals for the Insane and similar separate institutions. The Sisters believed that a psychiatric unit within a medical setting would promote early treatment and lessen the likelihood of long-term psychiatric care for many patients. Physicians, however, were not yet open to the idea. Over the next years, the neurology section cared for an increasing number of psychiatric patients, and Sisters offered their assistance. The neurology section's 1944 Annual Report notes: "The Sisters, especially Sister Domitilla, have come to our rescue in offering suitable quarters and trained nursing personnel for our psychiatric patients. We are indeed grateful for this offer of help." In 1946, the "Section of Neurology" changed its name to the "Department of Neurology and Psychiatry," and the next year Mayo instituted the

Department of Psychiatry. Not surprisingly, the Sisters warmly welcomed the new department to Saint Marys Hospital.

In their resolve to incorporate medical advances, Mayo physicians and Sisters were of one mind. This commitment, which required enormous adaptation, sacrifice, and teamwork, recalled the early days of the Doctors Mayo and founding Sisters. Like their predecessors, physicians and Franciscans in 1945 shared an overriding goal—to save patient lives and serve suffering humanity.

As agents of change, the Sisters were a paradox. Throughout the war, like other Americans, they prayed for their country and gave thanks for victory. Unlike other Americans, the war left their lives relatively unchanged. In truth, the Sisters at Saint Marys Hospital had more in common with European nuns of the 6th century than with fellow Americans in 1945.

American Catholic culture of the 1940s and 1950s had not changed appreciably since the country's founding. In the typical large Catholic family, it was an honor when a daughter joined a religious order. At the beginning of the 20th century, almost 50,000 women belonged to American religious orders; 50 years later their numbers peaked at 200,000. Sisters served a wide spectrum of the Catholic population; they were founders and operators of colleges and hospitals, diocesan schools, orphanages, and homes for the elderly and destitute.

"For over two hundred years," notes historian Dolores Liptak, "U.S. Catholic women have enthusiastically entered religious life. There is no movement in modern Church history, in fact, that can rival this vocational phenomenon in numbers, scope, variety of structures, or degree of accomplishment . . . Yet the story of these women and their corporate mission has largely been left untold . . . Indeed, it is safe to say that the Catholic scholarly community has been very remiss in portraying the role of women religious and its significance in the creation of the U.S. Catholic Church."

If the general public has little knowledge about the contribution of Sisters, they know even less about the women themselves. As a framework for understanding the life of Saint Marys Hospital Sisters, the next pages provide a brief general background of religious life. It is important to note that this summary covers an historical period that begins in 529 A.D. with the founding of monasticism and ends with the Second Vatican Council, 1962-1965.

Sisters entered religious life as young women for the love of God. Their attraction to the lifestyle was something of a mystery—even to themselves. For some, Sister teachers and nurses often served as models. For others, becoming a Sister was not their first choice, but life experiences and reflection changed their minds. Prayer and counsel with trusted persons guided each woman's decision. Jesus Christ was their model and inspiration. On faith they followed a 1,400-year-old tradition of men and women who dedicated their lives to God within the Church. Sisters took vows of poverty, chastity, and obedience and lived them out in an ordered regimen of prayer and good works. Over the centuries, external monastic structures changed and new congregations emerged. Religious life, however, was essentially the same in 1945 as in 529, when Benedict of Nursia founded western monasticism at Monte Cassino.

Rochester Franciscans, like most congregations, were not monastics, that is, they were not attached to an autonomous monastery where they lived, worshiped, and worked. However, like every religious congregation throughout the world, their Rule contained strong elements of early Benedictine monasticism, namely, communal prayer, meditative silence, and a cloistered environment.

Monasticism had its roots in early Christianity. Persecution under Roman Emperors marked the first three centuries of Christianity. It was the age of martyrs, when Christians died rather than give up their faith. Roman persecution flourished until 312, when Emperor Constantine had a remarkable experience. Riding through France with his army, Constantine looked up and saw a cross of light with the inscription, "In this sign conquer." Going into battle with the odds against him, he put a Greek monogram of the first letters of the name of Christ (CHR) on his standards. Constantine won the battle, became a Christian, and Christianity became the state religion—with far-reaching consequences—"To change the religion of the Roman Empire was to change the world."

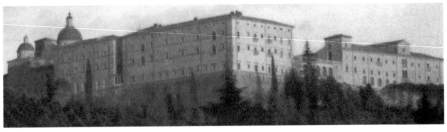

The monastery of Monte Cassino, founded in 529 A.D. by Benedict of Nursia, who wrote the Benedictine Rule. (From http://www.catholic-forum.com/saints/ncd05562.htm. Used with permission.)

Constantine made another decision of major importance. He moved the capital of the Roman Empire eastward from Rome to Greece. The Eastern Empire, well defended militarily, had a larger population and stronger economic and cultural base than its western counterpart. Constantine built a new capitol, Constantinople, now Istanbul, on the site of the Greek city of Byzantium. His geopolitical decision divided Christendom into east and west, with a Latin Church based in Rome led by the popes and an Eastern or Byzantine Church lead by the patriarchs. Strategically, Constantine's decision left Rome, and the entire west, vulnerable to increasing attacks by barbarian hordes.

Christian monasticism began in the civilized society of Greece in the 4th century, and Eastern Christendom provided 600 years of peace and prosperity for its development. Historian Kallistos Ware describes monasticism as a "fresh expression of the ascetic spirit present in Christianity from the start." Earlier, hermits of Palestine and Syria and groups of Christians in Egypt withdrew to the desert in search of a purified lifestyle. It was no coincidence, according to Ware, that monasticism emerged as Christians took privileged positions in society. The age of martyrs was over, and monastics kept the spirit of self-sacrifice alive, "reminding the church at large, that God's kingdom is not to be identified with any earthly realm."

Two centuries later, monasticism began in the west when the Roman Empire was awash in war, barbaric atrocities, and civil chaos. Germanic tribes from Asia and the steppes of Russia in the east infiltrated and ravaged the militarily vulnerable Roman Empire. After deposing the emperor and sacking Rome in 476, barbaric tribes devastated populations across Europe and the British Isles. They destroyed the Roman infrastructure and decimated the empire's economic, social, and cultural resources. Without Roman governance and law, all western society was in turmoil. Only the Church offered continuity and stability for Christians and non-Christians alike.

Barely 50 years after the fall of Rome, Benedict of Nursia established a monastery at Monte Cassino in southern Italy. His original intention was to found a religious order for men, but his twin sister Scholastica persuaded him to also found an order for women, which she headed. "The object of their endeavor," writes historian Joanne McNamara, "was to mold each individual into part of the whole and create for each person a life constantly informed by prayer." Like the earliest Christians, they held everything in common; nothing was considered anyone's personal property. "Love of God was love for the sick, for the poor, and for the traveler." The purpose of monastic life, according to Benedict, was "to honor God by worship and to benefit the community by prayer." Benedict discouraged austere penitential religious practices and encouraged lives of balance and moderation. Monasteries were autonomous and self-sustaining; monks and nuns worked in the fields and did other manual labor. The essence of the Rule of St. Benedict is "ora et labore" (in Latin: "pray and work").

The pressing needs of society called monastics out of their cloisters in the west. Missionaries, trained in monasteries, converted the Germanic peoples. Monks and nuns civilized indigenous peoples, restored culture and learning, preserved records, and produced beautiful manuscripts of Scripture and the classics. Indeed, monasticism shaped the religious, social, and cultural context of medieval society.

For eight centuries Benedictines were the only religious order in the Catholic Church. Over time, Rome centralized monastic jurisdiction and regulated its development in a Vatican office. As new religious orders like the Franciscans emerged, this office regulated them as well. Given monasticism's extraordinary stability and contribution, the Benedictine rule became the norm. Communal prayer, meditative silence, and a cloistered living environment were standard practices of every religious congregation, regardless of its founder and purpose.

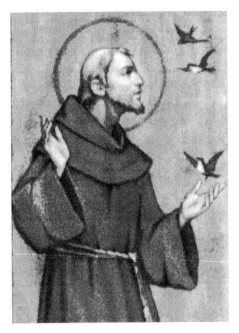

St. Francis of Assisi, 1182-1226, made poverty and love the centerpieces of Christian living and gained thousands of followers. (From http://www.catholic-forum.com/saints/stf01011.gif.)

In the 13th century, Saint Francis of Assisi founded a new religious order that addressed critical needs of the time. The Church had lost touch with the laity, clerical abuses abounded, and heretical movements gained recruits. Franciscans ministered outside the confines of a monastery. Francis and his followers settled in a rural chapel outside Assisi. According to historian Dominic Monti, "they spread out in small bands through central Italy, devoting themselves to contemplative prayer, working as day laborers and preaching, calling all to conversion by their word and example."

Francis made poverty and love the centerpieces of Christian living and gathered thousands of followers. The order's popularity was due partly to Francis' personality, his infectious enthusiasm, gaiety, and love. The basic principles he gave his followers were to help others by working in the world, preaching the gospel, and caring for the sick and suffering. In all, St. Francis founded three Orders: the First Order for men; the Second, with Clare Offreduccio of Assisi, for contemplative women; the Third Order for men and women, laypersons and religious sisters, priests, and brothers. The Third Order evolved into two distinct ways of life: the Secular Franciscans for the laity and the Third Order Regular for religious congregations. Rochester Franciscans followed the Third Order Regular Rule.

As noted earlier, the summary of religious life above applies to the historical period from the founding of western monasticism in 529 to the end of the Second Vatican Council in 1965. Broad pronouncements of the Second Vatican Council radically changed the Church and religious life. Future chapters will attest to its influence on Saint Marys Sisters and on the hospital as an institution. No one in 1945, or even 1955, would have anticipated this historical shift. Catholic scholar Sandra Schneiders wrote about the impact of the Second Vatican Council: "I want to focus on the extraordinary experience of women religious since the close of Vatican II. In effect, Religious in those three decades made the passage from the Middle Ages to postmodernity, which took western humanity seven hundred years to accomplish. The transition through which they have passed is unprecedented in scale, scope, depth, and radicality, and the disorientation of this period can only be understood in the light of that fact."

In the mid 1940s, 75 Sisters served at Saint Marys; two of them, Sisters Sylvester Burke and Constantine Koupal, were among the hospital's six original Sisters. For many, Saint Marys Hospital was their first assignment and they stayed 30, 40, or 50 years. The Doctors Mayo and physician colleagues were like family to them, as were all the hospital employees. Sisters' loyalties went deep for the persons and institutions of Saint Marys Hospital and Mayo Clinic. It may seem curious, then, that their interactions were limited to professional duties and formal events, such as graduations and hospital celebrations. Such restrictions, however, were part of the cloistered life they had chosen—"to be in the world, yet not part of it."

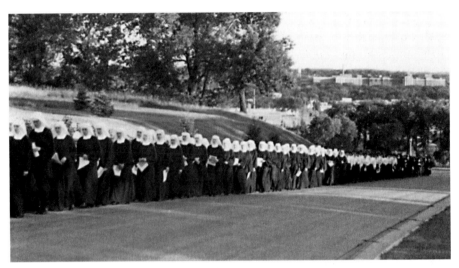

The Sisters of St. Francis in procession at Assisi Heights in 1963. (From A Century of Caring: 1889-1989. Rochester, MN: Saint Marys Hospital, 1988, p 89.)

Sisters shared a common dining room and community room. They used available rooms throughout the hospital as bedrooms until 1941, when the Francis Building was completed. Patients were moved to the new facility from the old 1912 building, near the chapel, and it became the Sisters' convent. They rose at 4:55 each morning and began the day in chapel with communal prayer, a version of the monastic Divine Office, followed by Mass. Sisters prayed as a community again in the afternoon at 2:00 or 5:00, depending on their assignments. Their day ended at 7:30 with Night Prayer, which began a period of strict meditative silence that lasted until the close of Morning Prayer the next day. They followed this schedule seven days a week until the 1950s, when they received one day off a week.

Though their daily schedule incorporated Benedictine monastic practices, the Sisters were Franciscans in name and spirit. They placed high priority on Franciscan hospitality, expressed in a variety of ways—annual ice cream socials, Christmas coffees, barbecues, and anniversary celebrations for Saint Marys Hospital employees. Sisters baked surprise birthday cakes, brought coffee to bedside watchers in the middle of the night, prayed with fearful patients, comforted anxious family members, and checked on patients "just one more time" to let them know that the Sisters would be with them through the long night until morning. On holidays, Sisters always worked a full shift so employees could be home with their families.

Love of beauty and God's creation, qualities attributed to St. Francis, expressed itself in art and architecture at Saint Marys. From the institution's beginnings, Sisters invested earnings to make the hospital more inviting and homelike. As their earnings grew, new hospital additions used architecture, design, and landscaping that "create relaxing and healing images for patients, visitors, and staff." Courtyards with flowering trees and statuary provide peaceful spots for reflection. Exquisite objects

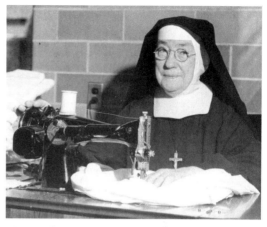

Sister Sylvester Burke, one of the hospital's founding Sisters, was for many years nursing supervisor for William J. Mayo, M.D. She enjoyed working in the operating room's mending room in later years (pictured here in the 1950s). (From A Century of Caring: 1889-1989. Rochester, MN: Saint Marys Hospital, 1988, p 72.)

of art and window vistas of nature from patient rooms renew soul and body.

According to Karen Moxness, "If you were ever in need, the Sisters were there for you." Karen, a clinical dietitian, served at Saint Marys in a number of positions. She recalled an instance when an employee and her family lost their home to a devastating fire. "The Sisters went into action immediately—two or three took charge. First, they determined the family's needs, next, they got the word out to employees and others who could help. Then they set up a collection system and a temporary headquarters. It seemed like only a matter of hours, before the Sisters delivered clothing and household items to the family. Their help continued, but it was the Sisters' immediate response that probably helped that poor family when they needed it most."

"At times of crisis the Sisters were there for us." Charlotte Carey, nursing supervisor in the emergency room, will always remember the June night in 1978 when the Zumbro River overflowed and floods caused death, injury, and widespread displacement. "We were working as hard as we could to help hundreds of people who came to the ER. About midnight I took a minute to check the waiting room. What a surprise to see Sister Generose, then head of the hospital, with her sleeves rolled up, mopping the floor. All around her, scores of injured waited for medical help. It must have meant a great deal for them to have her there—I know it meant a lot to me."

"How does a Sisters' hospital differ from other hospitals?" Sister Domitilla asked hospital administration students from Iowa City in 1953. She answered her own question, "The chief differences are due to the fact that a Sisters' hospital is their home. In this hospital there are slightly more than 100 Sisters on active duty. Their period of service varies from 1 to 64 years. We have one Sister, Sister Sylvester, who has been here 64 years. She came the year the hospital opened and is still active a few hours a day. She was Dr. William Mayo's surgical nurse during his whole professional life. This is home to her as well as to all the other Sisters on duty here." Ever the teacher, Sister Domitilla gave the students an assignment, "On your way back to Iowa City tonight, you might like to speculate on how that fact affects hospital construction, organization, and hospital administration."

Sister Domitilla's question in 1953 prompted a 2005 response from Robert Blomberg, education administrator for Mayo Health System. "The Sisters did a good job of managing the white spaces on the organizational chart." Blomberg referred to Geary Rummler's systems theory of organization. Rummler studied uncharted ways of *how work really gets done*. "When you do that," he wrote, "you see what we've known intuitively all along: anything that touches the customer is a result of a myriad of complex cross-functional processes." The classic way to picture an organization is to show many independent functions, usually a hierarchy of boxes. Opportunities for improving organizations are not found in the functions, "but in the handoffs between functions . . . in the white spaces between the boxes of the organization chart. All too often, no one is managing this white space. Things 'fall between the cracks' or 'disappear into black holes.'"

Making the connection with health care, Blomberg noted, "Patient care doesn't just flow vertically in organizational boxes, but horizontally across boxes. From long experience, Sister Domitilla and the Sisters knew that communication and teamwork are essential for a high standard of patient care." Teamwork and communication were central to the contribution of Saint Marys' service departments, such as the laundry, dietary, and sewing room. From the hospital's early days, when Sisters rose at 3:00 a.m. to do the wash, Saint Marys operated its own laundry. For years the laundry was a dingy, small annex of the hospital. Too small, in fact, to accommodate large equipment needed to wash heavy loads within a reasonable time. The laundry operated 14 hours a day. Not surprisingly, the first postwar construction at the hospital was a new laundry.

Sister Sarah Hoffmann, for years in charge of the laundry, worked tirelessly alongside employees who numbered about 20 in the new building. Together they accomplished an enormous daily task. Each morning head nurses requisitioned linen and twice a day laundry men picked up soiled linen from the floors. Between 7:00 a.m. and 1:00 p.m., mountains of linen went into one of five automatic washers, the largest holding 650 pounds. Agitated 43 to 63 minutes depending on the soil, linens went through one or more suds, bleaches, rinses, and blue baths until they were "hospital clean and white." Large extractors and tumblers dried most of the items; bed sheets went to 8-roll ironers, equipped with an automatic sheet folder. Women in the central linen room put requisitioned items into designated baskets and men delivered them to the floors. On an average day, a bed sheet sent to the laundry in the morning would be returned that afternoon.

Patient or direct laundry, as it was called, was only part of the laundry's responsibility. Much of the department's work was indirect and served the entire hospital: employee and student uniforms; bed linens for student nurses and dietitians; physicians' coats and gowns, masks for visiting doctors; curtains, drapes, and blankets; dishtowels, table linen and tray covers.

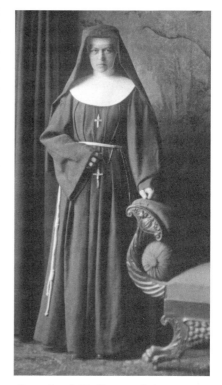

When asked about Sister Sarah, Sister Moira Tighe was quick to respond. "She worked harder than anyone I've ever known. I can still see her—physically strong, she wore sturdy shoes, and seemed to work all the time. She was quite reserved, spoke very little, but was always pleasant." Also known for her solicitous care of employees, Sister Sarah was particularly vigilant in the summers when laundry temperatures soared to 100 degrees. "She prepared gallons of an orange drink in the kitchen (I remember it always stained the pans). She insisted that employees drink large quantities and never forget to take their salt pills."

Sister Sarah Hoffmann, tireless super-visor of the hospital laundry. (From Saint Marys Hospital Archives.)

The sewing room worked closely with the laundry. Sister Angelica Osdoba and, later, Sister Ellen Klooster along with other seamstresses made all the hospital linen and took meticulous care of it. Sheets and linens were mended so carefully that their use extended far beyond most institutions and saved the hospital thousands of dollars.

In 1949, Saint Marys celebrated May 12, traditionally National Hospital Day, with tours of the hospital's service units. The *Rochester Post-Bulletin* quoted a hospital official, probably Sister Mary Brigh, who was in charge of the event, "These 'hidden services' are as much a part of hospital procedure as medicine and operations." Nearly 600 visitors toured the new laundry to see "the latest scientifically devised equipment." They also went to the large main kitchen in the Francis Building, where a menu of 3,600 meals a day is planned and executed. The assembly line tray service, the first of its kind in the country, served five trays per minute for medical patients. "Each tray is checked by a dietitian at the end of a conveyor belt before it is placed on a dumb waiter to be carried to the patient floors." One hundred full-time and 20 part-time employees prepared and served 110,000 meals monthly on trays for patients and employees on special diets.

As dietitian-in-charge of the kitchen from 1950 to 1957, Sister Moira worked with units responsible for specific units of food preparation. A Sister headed each unit, among them, Sister Bernadone Reining in vegetables and salads. Sister Bernadone and her workers carefully cleaned and prepared produce; some of the produce came from the Sisters' large vegetable gardens behind the hospital. Sister Ludovica pasteurized and bottled all of the milk, about 245,000 gallons annually, from Saint Mary's Farm. The Sisters' gardens and Saint Mary's Farm were vital to the hospital. Chickens and

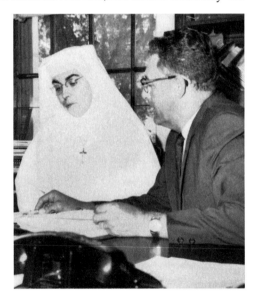

Sister Moira Tighe, in charge of the kitchen in the 1950s, later Director of Dietetics, works on a purchasing order with help from "Irv" Mullenbach, purchasing agent for Saint Marys Hospital. (From Saint Marys Hosptal Archives.)

livestock raised on the farm, along with fruits and vegetables from the gardens, provided Saint Marys with a regular source of fresh food of the highest quality for their patients and staff.

A young seventeen-year-old from Dickinson, North Dakota, Anna Jahner, later Sister Ralph, worked in the kitchen in 1937. The oldest of twelve children, Anna helped the family with her earnings from the hospital. As it turned out, Anna found more than a job at Saint Marys. Contact with the Sisters at Saint Marys and her three aunts, already Franciscans, inspired her to join the congregation. Years later, Sister Ralph enthusiastically recalled her work in the kitchen: "We had so much fun. The Sisters worked very hard and they kept us going too, but they were so good to us kids. If we did something wrong, they helped us do it right the next time. They were kind and understanding. You could tell them anything—they were always interested and that meant a lot to me, far from home."

"There were seven of us in that particular kitchen, five girls and two boys. Three of us were from North Dakota. We always got to eat with the Sisters in the kitchen. On feast days, like Saint Francis Day, Sister Antoninus [Windschitl] decorated the table beautifully. The food was special too. The way the Sisters treated each other impressed me. Never a sharp word, they respected each other. They were great models for me when I was assigned to head the kitchen at the College of Saint Teresa. I loved that work too and stayed for forty-eight years."

For the Benson family and other local families, among them, the Delaneys, the Reinings, and the Bowrons, working at Saint Marys was family tradition. Harry Benson, who retired in 1989, was the first staff member to work at the hospital for fifty years. Harry came to Saint Marys in 1939 and joined his sisters, Selma, Clara, and Mabel, who were already employed at the hospital. Harry suspected his sisters helped him get the job washing pots and pans in the kitchen: "My sister Mabel worked in the kitchen and I think she and my other sisters saw to it that I had a job where they could keep an eye on me. They and the Sisters of Saint Francis helped raise me." Harry's son, Carl, now works in the Security Department and carries on the family tradition.

Sister Moira had high praise for the Sisters in the kitchen, especially for their relationship with employees—with one reservation. "Some Sisters liked to give food to employees and made it difficult to manage the food supply. Sister Barnabas was in the bakery. She was a wonderful person, a superb baker, but generous to a fault. I remember pleading with her, 'Sister, you can't

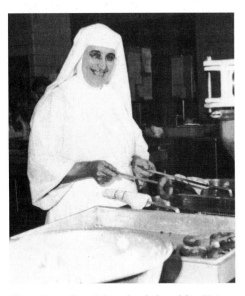

Sister Barnabas Schroeder, beloved by Sisters and employees, delighted in sharing her famous baked goods with others. (From Saint Marys Hospital Archives.)

give away any more pies.'" She'd smile that beautiful smile of hers and seemed to agree. Then, the next day, I'd see a young fellow coming out of the bakery with a towel over a tray—guess what?"

As practitioners of good employee relations, however, the Sisters in the kitchen could not be faulted, "for 25 years," Sister Moira went on to say, "our department had no union grievances. Those Sisters, and the way they treated employees like family, deserve much of the credit." In the early 1940s, employees in the dietary, laundry, housekeeping, maintenance, and power plant asked for labor union representation. Subsequently, they voted for a union and in July, 1946 Saint Marys Hospital signed a new contract with Local 515, United Public Workers of America, CIO. Dennis Hanson of Mayo Clinic's Labor Relations section later commented on the relationship of the Sisters with employees. "I've been impressed with the strong loyalty of employees for Saint Marys, whether they were union members or not."

The sacredness and dignity of the human person was almost bred in the Sisters' bones. This is the fundamental principle of a just society, according to Catholic social teaching. Rooted in Hebrew and Christian Scriptures, these teachings apply wisdom from writers as early as Augustine in the 5th century to contemporary issues. The principles of economic justice address labor unions: "The economy must serve people, not the other way around. All workers have a right to productive work, to decent and fair wages, and to safe working conditions. They also have a fundamental right to organize and join unions. People have a right to economic initiative and private property, but these rights have limits. No one is allowed to amass excessive wealth when others lack the basic necessities of life."

The dignity of the human person was Bishop Francis M. Kelly's theme for a 1941 presentation to Catholic nurses at a national meeting in St. Paul,

Minnesota. An acclaimed speaker, he was an untiring advocate for the elderly and chronically ill. Bishop Kelly urged faculty members of Catholic colleges and schools of nursing to include home nursing in the curriculum. About the same time, the bishop asked Sister Domitilla to consider home nursing services at Saint Marys Hospital. He probably knew his timing was good. Bishop Kelly was key to the Vatican's approval of the new medical building, then under construction. Somewhat reluctantly, Sister Domitilla agreed to establish home nursing services at Saint Marys. Her reluctance was no reflection on home nursing; rather, Sister Domitilla hesitated initiating a new nursing commitment when the hospital already faced a dire shortage of nurses.

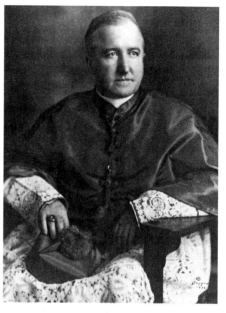

Francis M. Kelly, Bishop of the Diocese of Winona, an advocate for the elderly and chronically ill, enlisted help from the Sisters in this ministry. (Courtesy of the Diocese of Winona, Winona, MN. Used with permission.)

In September 1943, the *News Bulletin* announced Saint Marys Home Nursing Service: "Recently Saint Marys Hospital inaugurated a new service intended to bring to the sick, in their homes in need of nursing care, the services of a nurse. While the Saint Marys Home Nursing Service is a private agency sponsored and supported by the hospital, it has the approval of, and cooperates with, the Public Health Agency of Rochester. This service is rendered free of charge to all who may need it. Calls are accepted directly from the family, through the pastor of any church, the physician, the Public Health Agency, or the Seton Guild."

Sister Eymard Tracy, then supervisor of Saint Marys pediatrics department, became supervisor of home nursing. In preparation, she studied public health nursing at the Catholic University and worked with the Henry Street Settlement in New York City. Sister Eymard supervised the program for 41 years; notably, the program ended with her retirement in 1984. Sister Mary Lou Connelly, who worked with Sister Eymard for several months, recalled that she visited patients several times each week and taught family members how to care for them. Sister Eymard also supervised students in home nursing from the diploma, degree, and practical nurse programs.

Sister Eymard also spent much of her time caring for the mental, social, and spiritual needs of her patients. Her name was synonymous with home health care in the city of Rochester. William "Bill" Walker, who worked with Sister Eymard over many years, admired her as a person and enjoyed her company. "She could relate to persons from a wide variety of backgrounds—all in the interest of people helping people."

Sister Eymard was a great favorite with laypersons and had no shortage of willing volunteers for her projects. She initiated and supported a wide spectrum of programs, among them, Golden Agers, Seton Guild Crafts, Cronin Home for recovering alco-

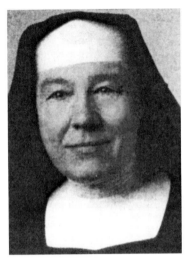

Sister Eymard Tracy inaugurated and supervised Saint Marys Home Nursing Service for 41 years. A formidable presence, she served on the White House Conference on Aging in 1960. (From Assisi Heights Archives.)

holics, Guest House for alcoholic priests and its auxiliary prayer group, St. Raphael's Guild. For her extensive contribution, Sister Eymard received city, state, and national recognition. The Rochester Exchange Club gave her the Golden Deeds award in 1958, Governor Orville Freeman appointed her to the first Minnesota Governor's Council on Aging in 1956 and in 1960 she was an official delegate to the White House Conference on Aging.

Richard "Dick" Edwards, administrator of Charter House, Mayo's retirement residence for seniors, knew Sister Eymard all his life. Reflecting on their lifelong association, he noted, "Long before people could even spell 'geriatrics,' Eymard was on the cutting edge. It's interesting that this has been my life work as well. Sister Eymard was a formidable woman, a handsome woman, who brooked no opposition. Figuratively, she carried a big stick and wielded great influence in the community."

Dick's mother, Mary Genevieve Clark, graduated with Sister Eymard from Saint Marys School of Nursing. "She and my mother did public health nursing long before it was commonly known in Rochester. They ran around town giving shots and doing good. From the time I could drive, it was my job to lug her around. Mother would say, 'Eymard has a box—go get it.' I'd drop whatever I was doing, no questions asked and deliver the box to some needy family. She worked with the folks who needed help but fell through the cracks. She was our version of Mother Teresa and everyone who was down and out found their way to Eymard."

During the war, as noted earlier, Saint Marys experienced a severe nursing and personnel shortage; after the war, when patient numbers soared, the employment crisis became even more acute. "Help Wanted" signs regularly appeared in the hospital's main lobby. Frequently, job applicants were family members of hospitalized patients. Desperately in need of workers, the dietary department hired them. Too often, however, when a hospitalized family member was discharged, these short-term employees took off their aprons, said a quick goodbye, and left fewer employees to prepare hundreds of meals.

The critical shortage of nursing staff forced Sister Domitilla to close 100 beds in August 1946 "for an indefinite time." Mayo hospital representatives, J. M. Stickney, M.D., and John M. Waugh, M.D., met with Sisters Domitilla, Mary Brigh, and Antonia and drafted a proposal for the Board of Governors. To lessen the duties of nurses, they proposed delegating specific duties, such as requesting tests, special examinations, and x-rays, to resident physicians. The Board approved the proposal and advised staff members in a bulletin.

Like Mayo Clinic, the Franciscan congregation stepped forward to help with the hospital's employment crisis. In the past, because of the need for teachers, the congregation assigned only one or two Sisters to Saint Marys each year. In 1947, the new mother superior, Mother Alcuin McCarthy, changed that practice and the *News Bulletin* carried the good news: "Fourteen new Sisters have come to Saint Marys Hospital this month. Seven of them will be students and seven are prepared to fill staff positions." Sister Jean Schulte (Sister Lea), assigned to study nursing, remembers the day she arrived at Saint Marys. "The Sisters gave us a wonderful welcome. Most of them were older and exhausted from years of responsibility. They were thrilled to see all of us young ones and we were delighted to be there."

A national crisis, the nursing shortage figured importantly in Sister Domitilla's decision to open a school of practical nursing. Practical nurses, trained in 1 year, would "care for patients under the guidance of registered nurses or physicians." Establishing the school was a bold step in its time. Practical nursing had skeptics among nursing leaders and graduate nurses. Indeed, at an earlier time Sister Domitilla probably would have been among them. Her continued commitment to nursing combined with administrative experience, however, changed her perspective. "In her view, nursing was not a profession unto itself, but one component of a team whose overriding goal was care of the sick."

Sister Generose was still a dietetic intern in 1947 when Sister Domitilla asked her to direct the practical nurse program. "I said I didn't know how I could be a director when I wasn't a nurse." Sister Domitilla then asked Rose Peturka, a graduate of Saint Marys School of Nursing with experience in this field, to become director. Sister Generose, who became co-director later, spoke about Rose Peturka: "She was a good, hard-working person, very patient with students and the students turned out well." Indeed, the entire program excelled and graduates served Saint Marys Hospital and other institutions with distinction.

Not long after celebrating the first graduation of the practical nurse program in January 1949, Sister Domitilla asked to be relieved of her assignment as administrator. The following December she became consultant for the congregation's four health care facilities: St. James Hospital in St. James, Minnesota; Mercy Hospital in Portsmouth, Ohio; St. Francis Convalescent Home in Denver, Colorado; and the Alfred Convalescent Home in Rochester. She also chaired two new and important building committees, one for a new motherhouse on Assisi Heights and the second, a major addition to the hospital, ultimately named the Domitilla Building. At her request, Sister Domitilla continued to teach basic sciences in the practical nurse program.

Sister Mary Brigh Cassidy, who would ably succeed Sister Domitilla as hospital administrator, wrote several excellent tributes to her predecessor. In a less formal piece, she described Sister Domitilla's contribution to the new motherhouse and hospital unit. "She had an unusual appreciation of beauty in structure and natural materials and both of these buildings will forever bear traces of her careful planning and sure instinct for what is right in design. She had a genuine interest and appreciation of art which was effective in resisting a human tendency to clutter up the place with non-essentials."

The recipient of many awards, Sister Domitilla was particularly touched by the tribute of Mayo colleagues presented in an illuminated scroll: "Members of the Board of Governors of the Mayo Clinic present this token of their esteem, of their high admiration for her wise administration, under which Saint Marys maintained and increased its position of pre-eminence in the hospital world, and of their gratitude for her sympathetic understanding, able counsel, and good humor when meeting problems which concerned the hospital and the Clinic."

Typically, Sister Domitilla typed her personal remarks in advance; in her droll way, she dubbed it, "The Scroll Moth Ball Affair."

"I accept your gracious tribute and high honor with mixed feelings of pleasure and embarrassment. I realize more keenly than any one else possibly can that the accomplishments you so generously ascribe to my efforts resulted from the encouragement and support of my superiors and the cooperation of my fellow-workers. As spiritual writers frequently say, 'Some of us are poor instruments, but in proficient hands.' I am deeply indebted to the Clinic as a whole, but especially to the men who were appointed to assist with some of the problems in hospital administration. They have never failed to be a source of strength and inspiration . . . In the name of Mother Alcuin and the Sisters, I accept and share this honor you have so graciously presented."

ENDNOTES

Page 71   Schneider CJ, Schneider D: *World War II: An Eyewitness History.*
                 New York: Facts on File, Inc., 2003, p 306.

Pages 71-72   Bordley J III, Harvey AM: *Two Centuries of American Medicine: 1776-*
                 1976. Philadelphia: W. B. Saunders Company, 1976, pp 385-386.

Page 72   New Operating Rooms Opened at St. Mary's. *Saint Marys Alumnae*
                 Quarterly Vol. XXIV, no. 4, October 1940, pp 14-15.

                 Saint Marys Hospital Annals. Development of operating rooms sec-
                 tion. "1947—Two rooms for urology and one for cystoscopy com-
                 pleted."

                 A Century of Caring: 1889-1989. Rochester, MN: Saint Marys Hospital,
                 1988, p 114.
                 The first post-anesthesia room was established at Saint Marys.

                 Grobe ME: *Development of Nursing at Mayo Clinic* [videorecording].
                 Rochester, MN: Mayo Foundation for Medical Education and
                 Research, 1993.

                 Annual Report, Neurology Department, 1944, Mayo Historical Suite.

Page 73   Interview with Saint Marys' Sisters. October 16, 2004. (Sisters Paula
                 Leopold, Pauline Brick, Vera Klinkhammer, and Antoine Murphy).
                 Impact of World War II at Saint Marys Hospital.

                 Stewart GC Jr: *Marvels of Charity: History of American Sisters and*
                 Nuns. Huntington, IN: Our Sunday Visitor Publishing Division, 1994,
                 pp 14-15.

Page 74   Chadwick H: The Early Christian Community. In: *The Oxford*
                 Illustrated History of Christianity. Edited by J McManners. Oxford:
                 Oxford University Press, 2001, p 61.

Pages 74-75   Ware K: Eastern Christendom. In: *The Oxford Illustrated History of*
                 Christianity, pp 131-132.

Pages 75-76   McNamara JK: *Sisters in Arms: Catholic Nuns Through Two Millennia.*
                 Cambridge, MA: Harvard University Press, 1996, pp 140-141.

Page 76   Cavadini JC: Monasticism. In: *Encyclopedia of Catholicism*. Edited by RP McBrien. San Francisco: Harper Collins, 1995, pp 883-888.

Monti D: Franciscan Order. In: *Encyclopedia of Catholicism*, pp 530-531.

Page 77   Stewart GC Jr: *Marvels of Charity: History of American Sisters and Nuns*, pp 33-34.

Schneiders SM: *Religious Life in the New Millennium*. Vol 1. New York: Paulist Press, 2000, p 100.

Pages 78-79   *A Century of Caring: 1889-1989*, p 73.

Page 79   Interview with Karen Moxness, November 19, 1998.

Self-Guided Tour, Saint Marys Hospital. Rochester, MN: Mayo Press, 1999.

Interview with Charlotte Carey, February 17, 2005.

Pages 79-80   Saint Marys Hospital Archives. Sister Domitilla's Presentation, May 28, 1953.

Page 80   Interview with Robert Blomberg, March 29, 2005.

Rummler GA, Brache AP: *Improving Performance: How to Manage the White Space on the Organization Chart*. Second edition. San Francisco: Jossey-Bass Publications, 1995.

Special report: Managing the White Space: The Work of Geary Rummler. *Training and Development* August 1992, pp 26-30.

Page 81   Interview with Sister Moira Tighe, May 12, 2005.

Pages 81-82   Interview with Saint Marys Hospital Sisters, January 29, 2000.

Page 82   *Rochester Post-Bulletin* May 6, 1949, p 5.

Whelan E: *The Sisters' Story: Saint Marys Hospital—Mayo Clinic 1889-1939*. Rochester, MN: Mayo Foundation for Medical Education and Research, 2002, pp 133-135.

Page 83   Interview with Sister Ralph Jahner, April 19, 2005.

                 Interview with Carl Benson, June 7, 2005.

                 Saint Marys Has Been More Than a Place to Work for Harry Benson.
                 Saint Marys Hospital Review **March 1989, pp 4-5.**

Pages 83-84   Interview with Sister Moira Tighe, January 25, 2005.

Page 84   *Saint Marys Hospital News Bulletin* **Vol. V, no. 7, July 1946, p 1.**

                 Interview with Dennis Hanson, August 28, 2003.

                 **Major Themes From Catholic Social Teaching: Economic Justice, p
                 3. Available from: www.osjspm.org/cst/themes. htm.**

Page 85   **New Home Nursing Service at Saint Marys Hospital.** *Our Sunday
                 Visitor* **October 24, 1943.**

                 Saint Marys Hospital News Bulletin **September 1943.**

                 Interview with Sister Mary Lou Connelly, November 4, 2004.

Page 86   Interview with William "Bill" Walker, November 11, 2004.

                 Interview with Richard "Dick" Edwards, September 14, 2005.

Page 87   Interview with Sister Moira Tighe, January 25, 2005.

                 Mayo Clinic Board of Governors' Meeting Minutes, August 12, 1946.
                 Recommendations:
                 A. Filling out requests for lab tests and x-rays
                 B. Placing calls for special consultation
                 C. Calling medical offices for representatives of the busiiness office
                 D. Filling out request for transfusions
                 E. Writing orders for tests, examinations, and special examinations
                 F. Cancellation of orders for tests, examinations, and special examina-
                    tions.

                 Sisters Missioned at Saint Marys. *Saint Marys Hospital News Bulletin*
                 August 1947, p 3.

                 Interview with Sister Jean Schulte, July 4, 2003.

A Century of Caring: 1889-1989, p 56.

Page 88   Interview with Sister Generose Gervais, April 12, 2005.

Saint Marys Hospital Archives. Sister Mary Brigh Cassidy papers.

Sister Mary Brigh: Sister M. Domitilla, O.S.F. *The Minnesota Registered Nurse* **23:83-84, 1950.**

Page 89   **Sister Domitilla's presentation "The Scroll Moth Ball Affair," Saint Marys Hospital Archives. January 27, 1950.**

CHAPTER 5

Collaboration

"$\mathcal{L}$ ong anticipated, long remembered," were the words of Edward
C. Kendall, Ph.D., at the 1949 announcement of the discovery of
cortisone. He wrote them on a souvenir photo for his colleague,
Philip S. Hench, M.D. Within the year, the two Mayo doctors received the
Nobel Prize in Physiology and Medicine for the discovery and use of cortisone. This scientific breakthrough presaged a new era of medical advances
for Mayo Clinic and Saint Marys Hospital. Collaboration among peers and
between the institutions was a key component in these accomplishments.

This and following chapters describe the decades from 1950 to 1980.
They open on a period of dramatic change and conclude with the retirement
of Sister Generose Gervais, the hospital's last Franciscan administrator. This
chapter examines the roots of collaboration among peers as well as within
each of the two institutions. It also describes the collaboration of nursing
Sisters as mentors for each other and as partners with Mayo colleagues.

Unprecedented numbers of young physicians discharged from the
armed forces began their medical careers at Mayo in the 1950s. At the same
time, unprecedented numbers of young women joined the Rochester
Franciscans and were assigned to Saint Marys Hospital. In this dynamic
context, Mayo and Franciscan values held firm. The welfare of each patient
continued to define the common purpose of Mayo Clinic and Saint Marys
Hospital. Collaboration, built on trust, was as important to the postwar
generation as it was to their predecessors.

The spirit of trust between the hospital and the Clinic was a conundrum
to outsiders. Richard Weeks, M.D., who came to Mayo in 1954, put it this

way: "Trust was a very important dynamic. Outsiders never understood the trust that existed between Mayo and the Franciscans." Early, formative experiences, in his opinion, built a foundation of trust. During his years as a resident in internal medicine, Dr. Weeks was on call at the hospital every third night. "As a young resident, I remember the night supervisors, who served as great resources for patients and physicians." Caring for patients in crisis, Dr. Weeks was indebted to Sister nursing supervisors for their willing help and seasoned expertise. In his words, "The Sisters were the backbone of the hospital."

Six night nursing supervisors, responsible for every patient in the hospital, served from 7:00 P.M. to 7:00 A.M. the next morning. Each supervisor kept in constant touch with her designated areas and personally visited critically ill patients. Years later, several of them looked back on their experience. "We had to be innovative and resourceful in crisis situations—to think through the patient's condition, consider possible responses, and sometimes make an immediate decision," commented Sister Jean Keniry. "When we came across something we didn't learn in nursing classes, our own Sisters were invaluable resources. They taught us from their years of experience; we could always count on their help."

W. Eugene Mayberry, M.D., began his internal medicine residency in 1956. Like Dr. Weeks, he was on call every third night and remembered the night nursing supervisors. "They were highly competent with vast responsibility. I particularly recall Sister Barbara Haag and how helpful she was to me as a young resident. Looking back, I believe it was the religious calling of the Sisters that made them such excellent colleagues for Mayo. Their lives were dedicated to the service of others and not to personal fame."

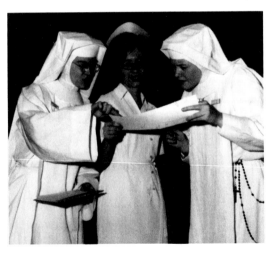

Sister Kathleen Lonergan (left), Marge Remick Connelly, and Sister Jean Keniry (right) avidly study a new report. (From Saint Marys Hospital Archives.)

Two young administrators began their careers at Mayo in 1950, David A. Leonard and Robert W.

Fleming. Unacquainted with nuns, Dave Leonard recalled his first impression of the Sisters: "They were highly respected, but everyone stood at some distance. Sisters came to the Clinic in pairs to do business and wasted little time in social interactions. There was a mystery about them and they weren't well known. Clinic people were deferential, but I sensed they weren't always sure how to approach them. In some ways, it must have felt cumbersome with no personal relationship to speak of, no entry beyond the basic politeness. Though few of us knew the Sisters personally, we were proud of the hospital and admired the selfless dedication of these women."

Expanded assignments increased Dave Leonard's contacts with Franciscans. Assigned to the personnel section of the Clinic, he worked with Sister Nora Logan, his counterpart at Saint Marys. "She was straightforward and a pleasure to work with in every respect." Dave Leonard came to know a great many Franciscans and played a central role at Saint Marys Hospital.

Major building projects at the hospital defined every decade between 1950 and 1980: the Domitilla Building in the 1950s, the Alfred Building in the 1960s, and the Mary Brigh Building in the late 1970s. Mayo's expanding clinical and surgical needs prompted the new construction. As early as the 1930s, Sister Domitilla initiated joint hospital planning committees for Mayo and Saint Marys. Joint committees offered members an opportunity to accomplish a common goal that served the interests of both institutions. In the process, communication increased and mutual trust deepened.

Bob Fleming, whose administrative career spanned 43 years, frequently served on committees with Saint Marys Sisters. An avid student of Mayo culture, he noted how the Mayo-Franciscan relationship contributed to the quality of patient care: "The Sisters and Mayo staff complemented and inspired each other with unique gifts and a single-minded purpose to serve the patients." Like Dr. Mayberry he recognized the complementary relationship of the two groups. Mayo colleagues admired the Sisters for their lives of service. In turn, their colleagues' compassion for patients, regardless of status or background, endeared them to Franciscans. For Sisters, care for each person, particularly the poor, was at the heart of the gospel they served.

Though the Clinic didn't flaunt its generosity, Sisters and others observed it in practice. Bob Fleming, for example, writes about an incident that happened shortly after he joined Mayo. Assigned to the business office, he learned to compute patients' bills and make arrangements for partial payments. "I still remember one Saturday morning waiting on a patient who seemed distraught. She informed me that her husband had died two months earlier, she had two children to care for, and she had just received a diagnosis of tuberculosis. She had limited financial resources and didn't know how she was going to arrange for the care of her children over the next few months while she underwent treatment. I discussed her situation with my boss, Mr. Vernon Tock, and asked if we should make an adjustment in the bill. He said that under the circumstances we should cancel the total bill. I informed her of the Clinic's decision and said that I hoped this would be of help to her and her family. She was deeply moved and appreciated the Clinic's compassion and generosity."

This story recalls the recommendation of Dr. William J. Mayo, noted earlier, during the Great Depression. "When it has been quite well demonstrated that an account is uncollectible, it is better to write the patient a pleasant letter enclosing a receipted bill, rather than engaging in any controversy or attempting to press collection indefinitely." Nearly 70 years later, when asked why Mayo tried to keep patient charges down, L. Emmerson Ward, M.D., responded, "People who are ill have so many concerns, we don't want to burden them unnecessarily with financial worry."

The remarkable story of cortisone again attests to the value of collaboration among Mayo peers as well as the two institutions. When Mayo's Board of Governors conveyed the Clinic's pride to the new Nobel laureates, Kendall and Hench deflected the praise. "In the whole world," said Kendall, "it could only have happened at the Mayo Clinic." Hench concurred, "Thanks, but the honor doesn't belong to me, I only wish Doctor Will and Doctor Charlie were here." Dr. Will had hired each of them: in 1914, at 28, Kendall became Mayo's first basic scientist; in 1921, at 25, Hench was the Clinic's first rheumatologist. Their praise for the discovery went to the Mayo founders and colleagues who taught them by word and example.

Edward Kendall, born and raised in Connecticut, received a Ph.D. in chemistry from Columbia University. His first scientific goal, to isolate the active hormone of the thyroid gland, brought him to Rochester, where he learned from the studies of Henry S. Plummer, M.D. Prior to his arrival at Mayo, Kendall had worked on this problem for over 3 years, at Parke, Davis and Company in Detroit, Michigan, and St. Luke's Hospital in New York City. Within his first year at Mayo, Kendall isolated thyroxin, the active hormone in the thyroid gland.

Kendall's research on the adrenal cortex, which led to the discovery of cortisone, began in 1930. Scientists had already determined that the adrenal

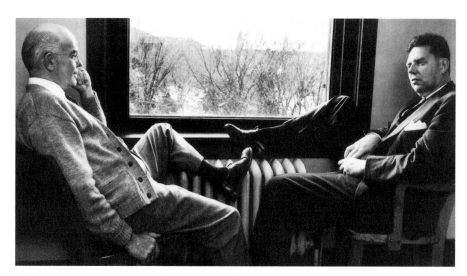

*Edward C. Kendall, Ph.D., a biochemist (left), and Philip S. Hench, M.D., a specialist
in rheumatic diseases (right), received the Nobel Prize in 1950 for research and clinical
studies that led to the discovery of cortisone. (From Milestones of Medicine [The
Eventful 20th Century Series]. London: Reader's Digest Association Limited; 1998.
p 124. Used with permission, Keystone/Hulton Archive/Getty Images.)*

cortex, the outer layer of the adrenal glands, produced at least one hormone
that was "necessary for life." Similar to his work on the thyroid gland,
Kendall's goal was to isolate the hormone. Unlike the discovery of thyroxin,
which he accomplished in less than 5 years, this project would require 18
years of uninterrupted research.

Later, Kendall reflected on his pursuit of the adrenal cortex hormone.
"What is the driving force," he asked himself, "that continues to exert
pressure during the five, ten, fifteen, or even twenty years" required for such
work? "Two components of the drive can be understood and are appreciated
by almost everyone. These are a love of whatever things are true and a
desire to create something. The scientist hopes to discover a small addition
to the accumulated truth of the ages and to create procedures that make
this revelation available to all. These hopes constitute a powerful drive that
is an inexhaustible source of strength."

"So modest, so nice, and so brilliant," wrote Hench in his journal after
meeting Kendall for the first time. Hench, on the other hand, was "a big,
hyperkinetic man who spoke incessantly." He taught by axioms, and lived
his own life according to two of them: "Work never hurt anyone," and "Go
after what you want." Colleagues said of him, "Long hours of work were

his way of life." In this respect, Hench and Kendall had a good deal in common. Reputedly, Kendall was "a man who celebrated Christmas Day, and indeed every holiday, in his laboratory." The drive and dedication of each one to his profession was essential to their common achievement.

Born and raised near Pittsburgh, Pennsylvania, Philip Hench received his medical degree from the University of Pittsburgh and came to Mayo as a fellow in medicine in 1921. Mayo leaders recognized Hench's intellect and energy and were also impressed by his early focus on the rheumatic diseases. They asked him to establish the first arthritis service and gave him good counsel: "He had the thoughtful supervision of Dr. D. M. Henderson, the personal advice of Dr. W. J. Mayo, and the help of Dr. Louis B. Wilson. Dr. W. J. Mayo advised Dr. Hench to 'spend your time in studying arthritis; if necessary, make yourself hard to find.'"

The arthritis service, which Hench headed, became a subspecialty of the Department of Medicine. Located in the old section of Saint Marys, the department had only recently become part of the hospital. The 1922 surgical pavilion added 300 new beds, which enabled Saint Marys to become both a surgical and medical hospital. Prior to this time Mayo medical patients were housed in several smaller hospitals downtown.

The medical department welcomed the opportunity to have patients in one location and to use the resources of Saint Marys Hospital. Leonard G. Rowntree, M.D., supervised fellows in medicine and clinical research. At Saint Marys Hospital, Rowntree created an adjunct department of medicine comprised of clinicians in several medical subspecialties. These clinicians, according to Mayo historian John L. Graner, M.D., were a loosely knit think-tank of physicians and researchers highly committed to their hospital services and research projects. As the only physician in the arthritis service, Hench was fortunate to have such colleagues in close proximity.

At the time, 3 million people in the United States alone suffered from rheumatoid arthritis. An incurable disease of the joints, its victims experienced crippling pain and other disabling symptoms, and no treatment existed that offered even temporary relief. As a world-renowned rheumatologist, Hench occasionally saw patients whose health improved under certain conditions. He hypothesized that something had prompted the secretion of a natural antirheumatic. In the late 1930s, Hench asked Kendall for help with his hypothesis.

"Whether Dr. Hench's power of persuasion or intuition on my part was responsible," Kendall recalled, "I became interested." Over the course of their talks, they decided that Substance X was probably an adrenal hormone.

"In January 1941 Dr. Hench and I had had a conference about arthritis. At the time both the chemical and the physiologic work were concentrated on compound E. The physiologic effects were striking and I was much encouraged . . . It was at that meeting that we decided to try the effect of compound E on patients who had rheumatoid arthritis."

Later the same year, the new medical building, now the Francis Building, opened with state-of-the-art laboratories and clinical research areas. Before Kendall and Hench could initiate clinical trials on "Compound E," however, World War II intervened. Hench had just enough time to help settle the arthritis service in its new quarters on the first floor of the Francis building before he left for the Army. After Hench's departure in 1942, his first assistant, Charles H. Slocum, M.D., became head of the section. That same year, Howard F. Polley, M.D., joined the arthritis service. Slocum and Polley staffed the arthritis section until Hench's return in 1946. Later, Slocum, Polley and nursing supervisor, Sister Pantaleon Navratil were responsible for the cortisone clinical trials.

During World War II, Kendall's laboratories focused on wartime research. When the war ended, Kendall resumed research on the adrenal cortex. He had the good fortune to work with a young chemist at Merck Laboratories, Lewis Sarett. Initially, compound E was available only in small amounts. Sarett discovered a way to synthesize "compound E" and make the hormone available on a broad scale. In August 1948, Kendall met Hench and informed him that "compound E" would soon be available. Not long after their meeting, Hench contacted Kendall about a patient with severe rheumatoid arthritis, 29-year-old Mrs. G., on whom he wanted to test the compound. Kendall agreed to obtain the necessary amount of "compound E. "

On September 21, 1948, Dr. Slocum gave Mrs. G. the first injection of "compound E." The next day, after a second injection, Mrs. G. remained virtually bedridden. On the morning of the third day, Mrs. G. found she could roll over in bed easily and began to regain her strength and appetite. Mrs. G. continued to improve, and within the week went on a 3-hour shopping trip in downtown Rochester.

After 7 months of trials, in April 1949, the team decided to release the results to their Mayo colleagues. Unobtrusively, they announced a presentation at the regular Wednesday evening scientific staff meeting. The meeting, packed with people, some of them perched on windowsills, included a film of the initial trials. The audience could see a patient, at first painfully and stiffly navigating several steps, then walking up and down the steps with ease, and finally running in place. The film made a dramatic, unforgettable impression. The audience gave Kendall and Hench a prolonged ovation.

Late in October 1950, when Kendall was in the barbershop across from the Clinic and Hench in Dublin on vacation, they received word of their Nobel Prize award. Tadeus Reichstein, Ph.D., of Switzerland was a third co-winner for his own important work on the adrenal cortex. In 1950, the Nobel Prize celebrated its 50th anniversary. At the formal ceremony, the king of Sweden personally presented the Mayo doctors with the Nobel gold medals. Each of them also received a monetary award of approximately $10,000 in Swedish kroner.

Emmerson Ward, M.D., joined the arthritis service about the same year Dr. Hench received the Nobel Prize. He was impressed with Dr. Hench's generosity in sharing his monetary award with colleagues, Slocum and Polley. Dr. Hench, who referred to Sister Pantaleon as "my invaluable colleague," established a travel fund for her to tour Europe and visit Rome for an audience with the Pope.

"We all admired Sister Pantaleon," Dr. Ward recalled, "she was balanced and efficient, with a good sense of humor." John Mayne, M.D., a rheumatology resident, later a consultant, also remembered Sister Pantaleon. "She was absolutely wonderful, ran the clinical areas superbly, and very ably assisted with clinical trials." Rheumatology patients, whose painful illness sometimes strained their good humor, usually responded to Sister Pantaleon's soothing, professional presence. Dr. Mayne recalled an instance when a patient was not so compliant. "This particular patient was often rude and abrasive. He developed a condition that required Sister Pantaleon to perform a difficult and distasteful procedure. In the process, the patient cried out, 'For Christ's sake, can't you stop?' Sister Pantaleon paused, turned to look directly at the patient, and said, 'Why do you think I'm doing this? I'm doing this in the name of Christ for you, sir.'"

Sister Pantaleon, formerly known as Elizabeth Navratil, like many Sisters at Saint Marys, first came to the hospital as a nursing student. Elizabeth, "Elsie," Navratil arrived in Rochester in 1926 from Silver Lake, Minnesota. As a student, daily encounters with suffering and death made a profound impact on her. Sister teachers were important role models. Within the year, Elsie and eight of her nursing classmates joined the Sisters of Saint Francis.

Native intelligence and good humor, combined with strong faith and high purpose, made Sister Pantaleon an excellent Franciscan candidate.

The rigors and discipline of religious training, however, tested the ideals and depth of resolve of new candidates. Those who persevered and received the approval of superiors made vows of poverty, chastity, and obedience. Prayer and sacrifice were their guiding principles in the spirit of Saint Francis, for the glory of God and service to others. Communal prayer, meditative silence, and a cloistered environment would frame their lives.

Sister Pantaleon served at Saint Marys from 1930 to 1955. She and her peers weathered the hardships of the Great Depression and bore the burden of shortages during World War II. Worn out from years of limited staff, they were overjoyed in 1947 when 14 young Sisters joined them at Saint Marys.

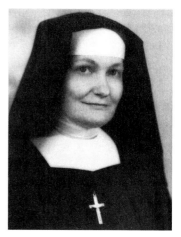

Sister Pantaleon Navratil, nursing supervisor for clinical trials that led to the discovery of cortisone. (From Saint Marys Hospital Archives.)

The young Sisters' religious training eased adjustment to the new environment. Religious practices they learned as novices were identical to those at Saint Mary's convent; indeed, they were the same in 1947 as the day the hospital opened. These practices and the values they represented linked Sisters together in a common life and mission. An ongoing challenge for Sisters, young and old alike, was setting aside personal interests in service to the common good. The spirit of sacrifice, a striking characteristic of Saint Marys Sisters, was essential in lives dedicated to serving others.

The years 1945 to 1965 were a watershed time for the Franciscan Sisters; unprecedented numbers of young women joined the congregation. World War II and its aftermath sparked a religious revival that swept the country. Although the movement quickly ebbed, choices of religious vocations continued strong through the 1950s and into the early 1960s. The Rochester Franciscans, for example, experienced a 32% increase during the 10-year period beginning in 1952, bringing their total membership to 955. The numbers of Sisters assigned to Saint Marys increased significantly during this period. Some served in hospital support areas; the majority, however, were in nursing.

The older Sisters made an immediate impression on Sister Barbara Haag when she arrived at Saint Marys. "They were gifted, hard-working women who hardly stopped from five in the morning until nine at night. Twelve-hour shifts were the norm and Sisters kept going if a new building needed cleaning or some emergency arose." During Sister Barbara's first years at Saint Marys, a Sister from the teaching ranks was assigned as superior, presumably to get the hospital Sisters in line. "The Sisters largely ignored her—they were very much their own persons. No one was going to tell someone like Sister Gertrude [Gaertner] not to get up in the middle of the night if a patient on her GI floor needed her. As night supervisor, I met Sister Gertrude more than once, caring for a desperately ill person at two or three in the morning."

Sister Generose, then assistant hospital administrator, was religious superior of Saint Mary's convent from 1954 to 1960. She was, for many young Sisters, a cherished, sustaining presence. Sister Generose drove the seven-passenger Cadillac, a gift from the Mayos, to the motherhouse every August. Young Sisters just out of the novitiate and assigned to Saint Marys Hospital waited for Sister Generose at the front door. Sister Rogene Fox was in her first group. "Sister Generose showed each of us to our rooms and made it a very personal experience, very welcoming. She was a wonder. As young Sisters we'd meet with her monthly and she'd talk with us about the vows, about spiritual life, about prayer. I don't know where she found the time to prepare for all of this, but she did and it was a wonderful experience for each of us personally. It helped bond us as a group."

Sister Mary Lou Connelly (Sister Leota) remembers the day in 1956 when she went to Saint Marys. "Ten of us piled in the Cadillac—excited and a little scared—we had a lot to learn. Sister Generose and the other Sisters taught us important lessons. Saint Marys was our hospital, our home, we owned it, it was our responsibility. Patients trusted us to give them the best care in the world. We were responsible for them 24 hours a day."

"I learned the value of fidelity, hard work, and community from Sister Digna in housekeeping, Sister Barnabas in the kitchen, Sister Julié in nursing. It was a hidden life of service. The work was unrelenting, you never went to your room to rest during the day. Yes, it was difficult, but I loved it—I liked caring for patients, teaching student nurses. I liked pitching in and helping out—and I've had good friendships among the Sisters. I've lived at Saint Marys for fifty years," Sister Mary Lou strongly affirmed, "and I've never wanted to leave."

Nursing historian Mary Ellen Grobe notes that the Rochester Franciscans began as a teaching order. These origins, in her opinion, "influenced their approach to developing caretakers for the hospital." When the Sisters needed additional nurses for Saint Marys in 1906, Sister Joseph established Saint

Marys School of Nursing. In the 1930s, as noted in chapter 2, Sister Domitilla presciently recognized that future nursing leaders would need a baccalaureate education. She designed a prototype for a Bachelor of Science in Nursing. Subsequently, Saint Marys School of Nursing and the College of Saint Teresa collaborated on the program. Under Sister Ancina, the baccalaureate nursing program went forward and became the standard for Sisters preparing for nursing leadership at Saint Marys Hospital. This achievement and its counterpart at other academic institutions, raised the educational level of nursing.

The emphasis on education at Saint Marys extended beyond formal programs and into the daily practice of patient care. Generations of Sisters and lay colleagues taught and learned from each other at the patient's bedside. They followed the apprenticeship method, which combined actual work experience with related instruction. As a model, it fostered a mentoring relationship and blurred traditional classroom barriers of teacher and pupil.

The majority of new Sisters were students in the baccalaureate nursing program. They worked on the floors at night and took collegiate classes during the day. "Our lives were simple," recalled Sister Rogene, "we worked, studied, prayed, and slept—it went something like this. We worked the night shift and went to 7:00 A.M. Mass. After breakfast, we slept for a few hours until we went to classes that began at 1:00. Later, we went to Vespers in chapel and studied whenever we found the time."

"It was an enormous responsibility as students to be in charge of a floor," recalled Sister Marilyn Geiger. "We looked to our Sisters for help and they were always there for us." Sister Barbara Goergen agreed, "Without their support and wisdom, it would have been much more difficult. When I became more experienced, I tried to do the same for others."

Student Sisters fondly remembered Sister Colleen Waterman, then night supervisor. "She made us breakfast every morning when we came off nights. It gave us a chance to wind down, to share experiences and laugh at each other—and ourselves." When reminded about all the breakfasts she made, Sister Colleen dismissed the compliment, "Oh, that was nothing, I remember what it was like as a student—if I hadn't made breakfast, they wouldn't take time to eat."

"I was thrilled to be in charge of a unit at night all by myself," recalled Sister Cashel Weiler, "but that confidence was buoyed up by the Sister in charge of that section of the hospital . . . These Sisters were always prompt to come. They never belittled one of our questions. They helped bring instruments and medications that were not ordinarily needed on one's unit. At the same time, they brought the invisible medicine of support and the nourishment that helped us grow as professional care givers. They seemed not only interested in the patient receiving prompt and excellent care; they were equally interested in each of us and in our development as young nurses."

After graduation, Sisters were typically assigned as head nurses. Relatively inexperienced, they relied on Saint Marys outstanding lay nurses for help and guidance. When Sister Jean Schulte became head nurse on third Francis, she was grateful to have Jean Dawson as her mentor. An exemplary nurse with vast experience, Jean invested her gifts and energies in guiding the new head nurse. Both resourceful women, they developed innovations that served patients well. Among these innovations was a variation of the team nursing model, noted in chapter 3, developed by Sister Antoine during the nursing shortage of World War II.

As head nurses, Sisters trained nursing students assigned to their floors. The vast majority of nurses caring for patients at Saint Marys at that time were students. After a 6-month probationary period of learning, observing, and practicing nursing techniques, every student nurse worked regular hospital shifts. Guided by nursing supervisors, students learned nursing by caring for patients.

Sister Faith Huppler, head nurse on third Domitilla, recalled her work with students. "I accompanied the physician consultant and residents on patient rounds every morning and reported on the status of each patient to the physicians. At the patient's bedside, the consulting physician taught residents through example and questions. I gained helpful patient information and insights on rounds and shared them with student nurses," Sister Faith noted. "Working with four or five students on a shift, I monitored their work and offered instruction as needed. Before a student went off duty, we visited her patients together. I assessed the quality of the patient's care and made suggestions for improvements. This was a teachable moment that students did not easily forget."

When Sisters recounted nursing experiences of the 1950s and 1960s, they spoke of the hours spent on sterilizing instruments and other items. "Every instrument, every bedpan, cotton balls, anything that touched a patient had to be sterilized," remembered Sister Dora Medina. "We used an autoclave, a device that steams items at high pressure. After long days with patients, I remember spending hours at night sterilizing bedpans and preparing equipment for the next day. We used items many times over before we threw them away. Rubber gloves were washed, powdered, and put in newspapers before they went into the autoclave. We made our own cotton balls, thousands of them, and sterilized them."

Sister Dora, a legend in her own time, was nursing supervisor of the 50-bed obstetrics ward for 20 years. Unlike most Rochester Franciscans, her roots were not in rural Minnesota, but rural Colorado, from a family of 13 children. Tragic loss at an early age had a profound influence on Sister Dora. "My carefree adolescent life ended when I was fifteen. That year my mother passed away in childbirth and great changes came over our family. At that time nine of us were school age and three were too young to attend school. At the funeral and wake, relatives and friends of the family offered to adopt some of us, especially the small ones. But, dad's response was final, 'No, thank you, we will all stay together.'

"Everyone had to sacrifice. Dad decided I would stay home with the youngest three until my older sister graduated from high school. My day was full caring for the children, doing the family laundry, baking enough bread for our meals plus extra loaves for all the lunch pails. When the older children came home from school they each had a job to do. The boys did the farm chores and the girls helped with cooking and ironing. After a year at home, I went back to school, graduated, and went away to study nursing. While I was a nursing student, I was inspired to enter a religious community. I became a Rochester Franciscan and soon a registered nurse.

"Rick [Richard S.] Sheldon, M.D., . . . worked with Sister Dora in obstetrics for 15 years. He recalls returning to the floor from the emergency room in the middle of the night and hearing Sister Dora's habit swishing as she walked the halls, making sure the patients had what they needed. 'She insisted on being available. She wanted to serve patients. She would help any way she could.'

"'She was a model for all nurses—for all of us," says Dr.

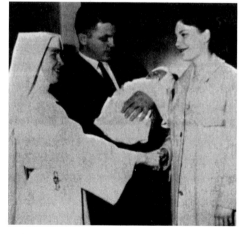

Obstetrics nursing supervisor, Sister Dora Medina, "a model for all nurses," says good-bye to new parents and their first baby. (From First year of classes educates 139 couples for parenthood. Saint Marys Hospital News Bulletin, June 1962;21:1.)

Sheldon. "Whenever the ward became busy with obstetric deliveries, admissions of threatened miscarriages, or there were illnesses among the staff, she was 'onboard' providing extra staff, serving as surgical assistant in the operating room, or following patients in the labor rooms while other nurses were occupied with other duties. She was always aware of the condition of ill patients on the floor, to provide progress reports if one of the staff would call from the Clinic or home about their patients.'"

In 2002, Dr. Sheldon and his obstetrics and gynecology colleagues established a nursing scholarship in Sister Dora's honor. "The Sister Dora Excellence in Nursing Award" recognizes nurses who demonstrate outstanding abilities in patient care.

In the 1950s and 60s, Sister Dora's name, like Sister Samuel Reinartz before her, was synonymous with obstetrics. During the same period, several Franciscans served in pediatrics, among them, Sister Regina Monnig (Sister Gretta), Sister Kathleen Lonergan (Sister Nuala), and Sister Frances McManimon.

Sister Regina worked with John Kirklin, M.D., who introduced open-heart surgery at Saint Marys in 1957. Dr. Kirklin's contribution to cardiovascular surgery had far-reaching consequences for the medical center. Initially, most of the patients were infants and children, as open-heart surgery concentrated on congenital heart defects. Desperate parents brought their children to Mayo from across the globe as open-heart surgery was the last resort. Sadly, many of the first surgeries were unsuccessful and children died. Others sustained the operation, recovered, and went on to lead full lives.

"After open-heart surgery," Sister Regina recalled, "I routinely helped children walk down the hall. One day I was helping a little boy about five years old when his mother saw us and burst into tears. I was concerned about the mother's reaction and asked her if I could help. The mother smiled and said, 'These are tears of joy. I've never seen my little boy walk before today.'"

Sister Kathleen Lonergan, nursing supervisor from 1961 to 1964, spoke about the hardship of parents whose children came for heart surgery. "Typically, children arrived a month before heart surgery as they were carefully monitored for infection and other problems. Throughout this period, parents were not allowed to visit their children. Dr. J. W. DuShane, a man of great compassion, was in charge of the unit. I spoke with him about the situation and proposed that parents, masked to guard against infection, be allowed to visit their children twice a day for 30 minutes. To the joy of parents and children alike, Dr. DuShane agreed to allow the new practice."

Sister Kathleen recalled benefactors, often parents, who provided funds for services and events that enhanced the lives of the children. The unit, for example, established a children's library with the help of a noted Rochester educator, Helen Remley. Parties, too, added a lively note, such as a circus party in the summertime with a beloved clown; on Halloween the children dressed in costumes went through the hospital collecting tricks and treats. "We always had a large Christmas party," said Sister Kathleen. "Thanks to a benefactor, nurses chose gifts, not only for the patients, but also for the children of staff members and residents. Sister Frances and her students put on a Christmas play and one of the doctors was Santa Claus."

Sister Frances McManimon taught nursing arts in pediatrics to students in the 3-year and collegiate programs. "Nurses monitored the children very carefully, checking vital signs literally every minute when necessary. Occasionally parents would ask for a special duty nurse, but this was the exception as the nursing care was so highly regarded. Physicians immediately involved the nurses in caring for a child as well as the parents. They all worked closely together throughout the child's hospitalization. I was impressed by the physicians' sensitivity to parents and the care they took in explaining the child's illness, ongoing progress, and prognosis."

The south wing had private rooms for very ill children. Restricted visiting hours, always difficult for parents, did not apply in this area. "Little ones never complain or fight insomnia, nor are they afraid to die, they comfort their parents. 'Don't worry. God likes me,' said one child." Sister Frances recalled an incident when a little 3-year-old tried to console her mother. "The little girl could tell how badly her mother felt. She looked up at her mom with big blue eyes, 'Dod is dood to liddle guls. [God is good to little girls.]'"

Children came to Mayo for a number of specialized surgeries, orthopedic surgery among them. Anthony "Tony" Bianco, M.D., a pediatric orthopedist and father of seven, was the first Mayo surgeon to specialize in children's bone surgery. Dr. Bianco's patients, who ranged from tiny babies to teenagers, required surgery for scoliosis, rheumatoid arthritis, fractures, or congenital abnormalities such as clubfeet. Like other Mayo physicians, Dr. Bianco consulted with specialist colleagues, such as a neurologist for the diagnosis of a child's bone tumor, in treating his patients. He also worked closely with pediatricians and nursing staff on the unit about the child's on-going care. Dr. Bianco commented on his experience at Mayo. "What makes this such a good place to practice is that we have so much support. It's a team effort in the finest sense."

For the Sisters in pediatrics and their peers at Saint Marys, attending the needs of patients was an uncompromising responsibility. Whether in charge of a nursing floor or serving another area of the hospital, most of the Sisters worked separately from each other. Community times together offered a degree of balance in their lives. Visits over meals, summer picnics, and community parties were highlights. In their own words, "they got us through." Sometimes Sisters bent the rules; 10 or more, for example, met for years in a surgery office after Night Prayer. "It was a lifeline for us," recalled Sister Jean Schulte, "a place of 'no rules' where we could talk about whatever we chose and didn't feel constrained."

"We had one day off a week," Sister Rogene recounted. "Most of us were in charge of a floor, so we spent a lot of the day making out schedules for the staff. We had a special perk on our day off—we could sleep in and go to 8:00 Mass. After Mass, six or eight of us would take a frying pan, an electric toaster, a coffeepot, and all the food we needed, and go to the pergola for a picnic breakfast. We had great times and that's what got us through—we were young, everyone around us was working just as hard, we didn't complain."

Sister Cashel wrote about her student memories of Sisters prior to joining the Franciscans. "Sometimes in the evenings we sat on the hill that surrounded the Sisters' evening gathering place to listen to the laughter that rolled out of the window so contagiously." Humor definitely sparked the Sisters' recreation times. Not surprisingly, stories they told on each other often centered on how tired they were. If an incident happened in the solemnity of chapel, all the better. "Like the time Sister Pauline Brick fell asleep in chapel. She woke up when the altar bells rang and announced, 'Good morning, this is Sister Pauline.'"

Sister Cashel's description of nursing at Saint Marys seems appropriate in a chapter about collaboration. "Doctors and nurses were not adversaries . . . It is difficult to know if this was the way the Sisters worked, the way the doctors worked, or if it was the entire medical center that worked this way. The patient was always the silent 'mission.' Each of us was a link in the chain. One's success was always latched on to the work of someone else. It would have been unthinkable to say, 'this was my success alone' or 'I was

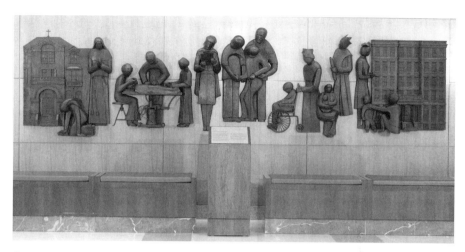

"Forever Caring," a 15-foot bronze tableau located in the Mayo Nurses' Atrium of the Gonda Building, depicts the history of Mayo nurses' commitment to the essence of their profession—caring for patients. (By artist Gloria Tew.)

the one responsible for that.' To have done so, even if it entered my mind, would have felt like treason. It was *always* our patients, our hospital, and our medical center."

ENDNOTES

Page 95   *Cortisone: Long Anticipated, Long Remembered; the Creation of Cortisone.* [Video script]. **Rochester, MN: Mayo Foundation for Medical Education and Research, 2000, p 8.**

Pages 95-96   Interview with Richard Weeks, M.D., August 5, 2004.

Page 96   **While Rochester Sleeps.** *Saint Marys Hospital News Bulletin* **January 1963, p 1.**

               Group interview with Sisters of Saint Francis: Sisters Jennifer Corbett, Marilyn Geiger, Barbara Goergen, Merici Maher, Regina Monnig, Carmen Sonnek, Helen Chatterton, Jean Keniry, Ancel Fischer, Elizabeth Gillis, Ruth Peterson, Moira Tighe, Jean Schulte, Mary Lynch, July 4, 2003.

               Interview with W. Eugene Mayberry, M.D., October 29, 2003.

Page 97   Interview with Robert W. Fleming, August 1, 2005.

Pages 97-98   Interview with David A. Leonard, July 18, 2003.

               Fleming RW: *Autobiography.* **Self-publication, 2002, p 57.**

Page 98   **Mayo Clinic Board of Governors' Meeting Minutes, October 21, 1931.**

               Interview with L. Emmerson Ward, M.D., August 1, 2003.

               Gastineau C: The Division of Endocrinology. In: *A History of the Department of Internal Medicine at the Mayo Clinic.* **Edited by JL Graner. Rochester, MN: Mayo Foundation for Medical Education and Research, 2002, pp 205-206.**

Page 99   **Kendall EC:** *Cortisone.* **New York: Charles Scribner's Sons, 1971, p 50.**

Pages 99-100   *Cortisone: Long Anticipated, Long Remembered; the Creation of Cortisone,* **pp 2-3.**

Page 100   **Conn D, Duffy J: The Division of Rheumatology. In:** *A History of the Department of Internal Medicine at the Mayo Clinic.* **Edited by JL Graner. pp 287-288.**

Graner JL: *A History of the Department of Internal Medicine at the Mayo Clinic*, pp 16-17.

Pages 100-101   Kendall EC: *Cortisone*, p 91.

Page 101   *Cortisone: Long Anticipated, Long Remembered; the Creation of Cortisone*, p 6.

Kendall (pp 124-125).

Page 102   Interview with L. Emmerson Ward, M.D., August 1, 2003.

Hench PS: A Reminiscence of Certain Events Before, During, and After the Discovery of Cortisone. Remarks made at the Centennial observation of the founding of St. Joseph's Hospital, St. Paul, Minnesota, May 16, 1953. (Saint Marys Hospital Archives.)

Interview with John Mayne, M.D., October 1, 2003.

Pages 103-104   Interview with Sister Barbara Haag, August 23, 2005.

Page 104   Interview with Sister Rogene Fox, September 5, 2005.

Interview with Sister Mary Lou Connelly, September 5, 2005.

Pages 104-105   Grobe ME: *Development of Nursing at Mayo Clinic*. [Videorecording]. Rochester, MN: Mayo Foundation for Medical Education and Research, 1993.

Whelan E: *The Sisters' Story, Part Two: Saint Marys Hospital—Mayo Clinic, 1939-1980*. Rochester, MN: Mayo Foundation for Medical Education and Research, 2007, pp 8-9.
The origins of the College of Saint Teresa's Bachelor of Science in Nursing (BSN) are described.

Page 105   Interview with Sister Rogene Fox, September 5, 2005.

Group interview with Sisters of Saint Francis: Sisters Jennifer Corbett, Marilyn Geiger, Barbara Goergen, Merici Maher, Regina Monnig, Carmen Sonnek, Helen Chatterton, Jean Keniry, Ancel Fischer, Elizabeth Gillis, Ruth Peterson, Moira Tighe, Jean Schulte, Mary Lynch, July 4, 2003.

Interview with Sister Colleen Waterman, January 3, 2006.

Pages 105-106   **Weiler, Sister Cashel:** *Sisters' Influence at Saint Marys Hospital* **(unpublished paper). September 1, 2005.**

Page 106   Interview with Sister Jean Schulte, September 9, 2005.

Pages 106-107   Interview with Sister Faith Huppler, November 7, 2005.

Page 107   Interview with Sister Dora Medina, February 8, 2005.

Pages 107-108   **Dr. Sheldon quoted in Finnamore H: Quiet Hero.** *Mayo Today* **November/December 2005, p 2.**

Page 108   *Sister Dora Excellence in Nursing Award.* **Mayo brochure, 2003.**

Interview with Sister Regina Monnig, September 14, 2003.

Pages 108-109   Interview with Sister Kathleen Lonergan, September 3, 2005.

Page 109   Interview with Sister Frances McManimon, September 5, 2005.

Pages 109-110   **The Physician at Saint Marys.** *Caring* **Fall 1977, pp 4-5.**

Interview with Anthony Bianco, M.D., September 29, 2003.

Orthopedic Surgery at the Mayo Clinic: 1910-1990. **Rocheser, MN: Mayo Foundation for Medical Education and Research, 1990, p 34.**

Page 110   Interview with Sister Jean Schulte, September 9, 2005.

Interview with Sister Rogene Fox, September 5, 2005.

Pages 110-111   **Weiler, Sister Cashel:** *Sisters' Influence at Saint Marys Hospital* **(unpublished paper).**

CHAPTER 6

Valued Relationships

*M*ayo colleagues agreed: Sister Mary Brigh is a "consummate business authority." Her peers, mostly men, described her with interesting variation. "Modest and reserved," wrote Victor Johnson, M.D., "she moved mountains while seeming only to be dusting a table." "Sister Mary Brigh was one of the few who could go one-on-one with Harry Harwick and win half the time," said an administrator. "She was a lady—a gentlewoman, with this quiet Irish 'chutzpah.'" At the Mary Brigh Building dedication, W. Eugene Mayberry, M.D., recalled a colleague's remark after a difficult meeting, "Sister wasn't even a gentleman!"

Her 22 years as hospital administrator gave Sister Mary Brigh her own perspective. "I have often thought, and sometimes said, I would hate to be a hospital administrator if I did not believe in God."

Sister Mary Brigh Cassidy's life story, even prior to her years at Saint Marys, was a rich and remarkable one. One of six daughters, Julia Cassidy was born in 1906 to Irish immigrant parents. Timothy Cassidy and Bridget Moroney Cassidy raised their girls on a farm near Eyota, a small town just east of Rochester. The Cassidy farm was not far from "Irish Ridge," home to Sister Joseph Dempsey, another daughter of immigrants and first administrator of Saint Marys Hospital.

Sister Mary Brigh remembered her mother as a lover of books who worked hard during the day and read voraciously at night. Julia also loved books and an English teacher once urged her to become a writer. During her senior year in high school, she was page editor for the former *Inter-County Press*, "going from hardware store to druggist to gather Eyota news." Julia, who seriously considered a career in journalism, was also drawn to teaching. Yet it was nursing that won her allegiance, thanks to the influence of Regina, an older sister and graduate of Saint Marys School of Nursing. Sister Mary Brigh said of nursing "it was a choice I never regretted."

Nursing students Julia Cassidy and Elsie Navratil were classmates. Elsie, later Sister Pantaleon, assisted with the discovery of cortisone. Elsie left nurse's training before graduation to become a Franciscan. Julia confided that she also "sensed a call to religious life," but put the choice aside. Instead, she went to Chicago and took a position as an obstetrical nurse. In 1928, the end of the "roaring twenties," Chicago beckoned many small town girls. A year later the stock market crashed and triggered the Great Depression. Julia found herself in a very different city. The country's largest manufacturing center, Chicago was hard hit by the Depression. Unemployment reached 50%—families starved for lack of food and the unemployed lived in city parks. "I do not know how it may have been in other places," one woman wrote, "but in Chicago the city seemed to have died. There was something awful—abnormal—in the very stillness of the streets."

The Chicago experience that beckoned with great promise became the crucible that changed her life. Stark, unrelenting poverty surrounded her. She described visiting patients in homes, "where people had nothing to eat and no heat." "My family had never been wealthy, but the idea of people living with so little was a kind of revelation to me." Julia found comfort in the poetry she liked to read and wrote some of her own. She also looked to her faith for strength and direction. In light of the Chicago experience, she reconsidered the call to religious life. "A vocation is a call from God. I didn't say 'no' the second time."

Julia returned to Rochester in the early 1930s to join the Franciscans. Sister Joseph and the other Sisters were delighted with her decision. Such news brightened a bleak time when hospital registrations sank 40% and the Sisters reluctantly reduced most of the lay staff. Julia served as night nursing supervisor during the congregational application process and entered the convent in 1935.

Sister Mary Brigh was 29 when she became a Franciscan. "In those days," she explained, "you were supposed to enter between 16 and 30. I still think about something a religious counselor told me then. He said, with my age and experience, he didn't know if I would be a better Sister or worse, but that I would be different."

Following the novitiate, Sister Mary Brigh spent the next 2 years in Winona and earned a baccalaureate degree in nursing at the College of Saint Teresa. She went back to the hospital in 1939, not long after the death of Sister Joseph. Returning to Saint Marys was akin to coming home. Doctors Will (William J. Mayo, M.D.) and Charlie (Charles H. Mayo, M.D.) and the founding Sisters "were not names but persons to me." "Saint Marys became part of me and although I went away for a few years at a time, I never really left it. Particularly, I never lost touch with its spirit of dedicated service to the sick, the desire to give the best that could be given with what was then available and to seek ways to make better, more cures possible in the future."

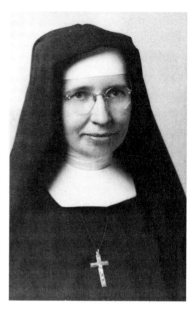

Sister Mary Brigh Cassidy, Administrator of Saint Marys Hospital, 1949 to 1981. (From Saint Marys Hospital Archives.)

Sister Mary Brigh's maturity, experience, and natural abilities impressed her superiors, particularly Sister Domitilla DuRocher. For the next 10 years she was on a fast track. After a short stint of teaching for Saint Marys School of Nursing, she went to the Catholic University of America in Washington, DC, for a master's degree in nursing. She returned to Saint Marys about the same time that Sister Domitilla created a personnel department. At Sister Domitilla's request, she organized the department and turned it over to a new director. She then went to the University of Chicago for a master's in business administration and finished in the spring of 1949. Later the same year, Sister Mary Brigh was appointed Saint Marys Hospital administrator.

After a decade of intense preparation and two years as hospital administrator, Sister Mary Brigh took a break. In 1952, she and former nursing classmate, Sister Pantaleon, went on a six-week European tour. As noted earlier, Sister Pantaleon received travel money from Dr. Philip Hench, who shared his Nobel Prize monetary award with valued colleagues. Not surprisingly, the Sisters used the opportunity not only for sightseeing but also for learning about European innovations in health care. Over the 6 weeks, they visited a score of hospitals on the Continent and British Isles—from Italy and France to Switzerland and Sweden and across the channel to England

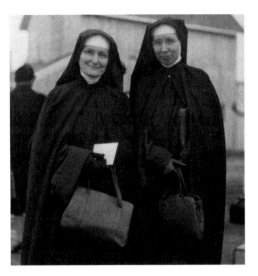

Sister Pantaleon Navratil (left) and Sister Mary Brigh Cassidy (right), old friends from nursing school, leave on a 6-week European tour in 1952. (From Saint Marys Hospital Archives.)

and Ireland. They returned to Rochester with new perspectives and renewed energies.

As a new administrator, Sister Mary Brigh was grateful for the unqualified support she received from Sister Nora Logan, who succeeded her as personnel director. Small in stature, Sister Nora was a powerhouse of focused energy. Sister Nora grew up in a large family on a farm near Rochester and graduated high school in the depths of the Depression. Instead of going to college, she took a business position to help the family financially. In her late 20s, Sister Nora entered the Rochester Franciscans. Her business experience served her well in congregational assignments, personnel director among them.

Personnel departments, well established in commerce and industry, were new to hospitals when Sister Nora became director. As noted in *Saint Marys News Bulletin*, the increasing size and complexity of modern hospitals "make organized personnel direction almost a necessity." The article went on to describe the new department. "The usual activities of the personnel department include the formulation of personnel policies and regulations, the interviewing and recommending applicants for positions, the training and induction of new employees, and an over-all program for promoting the interest and welfare of all employees."

Margaret Hermann, new to Saint Marys in the early 1950s, was delighted to serve as secretary to Sister Nora. Together they comprised the personnel department throughout the 1950s. "I wonder how we did it," Margaret commented. "Nothing was automated and I was responsible for time cards of all hospital employees. I did all the correspondence, interviewed every applicant, and sent the promising ones to Sister Nora." Margaret spoke highly of Sister Nora; "I admired her dedication and the way she treated people with honesty and compassion. She always told people what she expected of them. She looked them right in the eye and they knew she meant business. Many employees came to her with their problems and she always had time for them."

Sister Valerie Olson (Sister Katrine), the department's third member recalls the day in 1960 when Sister Mary Brigh asked her to go to personnel. "I worked in registration and information at the time. I was happy for the new assignment and enjoyed the job even more as the years went on." Sister Valerie became a skilled interviewer. With Margaret Hermann, she developed programs in recruitment and orientation as well as inservice training. The department grew in numbers and changed its name to human resources. Sister Valerie and Margaret were important links to the hospital's heritage.

Anne Purrington, who came to the department in 1980, worked with Sister Valerie and Margaret Hermann. "Their stories of the early years taught me about Saint Marys values. I learned how Sister Nora ran the department, how she treated people. I learned all the wonderful human stories that bring our legacy to life. Some call Human Resources the heart of the organization; we have an opportunity to make a difference in peoples' lives. This is what makes our work worthwhile—why we choose to serve in HR."

Two of Sister Nora's sisters followed her into the Rochester Franciscans. Sister Neal Logan, a nurse prior to entering the convent, worked in that field at Saint Marys and other congregational institutions. Sister Fidelis Logan, who served in education, had several assignments in Rochester Catholic schools.

"Sister Nora was a good listener," Sister Fidelis Logan observed. "It was probably her greatest gift. She was also compassionate with employees, especially those who might be having a hard time. The story of hiring Cyril Manahan is legendary. Cyril was a local farmer with a large family who came to see Sister Nora. 'I need an extra job,' he told her, 'farming isn't going well right now. I may not have special skills, but I sure know how to work.' Sister Nora was heartsick, 'Mr. Manahan,' she said, 'I'm sorry, the only job I have is for an elevator operator that begins tomorrow morning at 7:00 a.m.' Cyril paused, 'Thank you, Sister, I'll be here at 7:00 tomorrow morning.' Cyril Manahan went to work at Saint Marys the next day—and over the next thirty years held key positions in the facility department. He was hard working, dedicated to the institution, and a lifelong friend of the Sisters."

The Manahan family became part of Saint Marys—Cyril's wife Madeline Manahan worked at the hospital, as did most of the nine children. One of the girls, Kate, became a Franciscan with an abiding commitment to the economically poor. Sister Kate Manahan, who died in 1996, is remembered for many fine qualities, among them, the Irish wit she inherited from her dad.

Of all the people Sister Nora befriended, Ray Island seemed an unlikely candidate. Loud and brash with an irreverent wit, Ray was a Norwegian Lutheran from nearby Zumbrota. He was just out of alcohol treatment when he went to Saint Marys looking for work. "To tell the truth," Ray admitted, "I didn't want a job. I had to go through the motions to get unemployment insurance. So I wrote everything I ever did on the application—alcohol treatment three times, jailed for drunk driving, I didn't hold back. The waiting room was crowded. I was surprised when the office girl came over and said Sister Nora wanted to see me. I went to her office and the first thing she said to me was, 'This is the worst job application I've ever seen!' Then she looked me in the eye and said, 'Maybe I ought to have my head examined, but I'm going to take a chance on you.'"

"I was an orderly in surgery about a year when the mental health center offered me a job working with alcoholics. I went to see Sister Nora before I left and I guess we both cried a little. She told me if I ever needed a job to come back to Saint Marys. While I was working at the mental health center, Bob Morse [Robert M. Morse, M.D.] asked me to help him start Mayo's first alcoholism treatment unit. Over the years, I've worked with hundreds of alcoholics. They've helped me to stay sober and I hope I've helped them. But it was Sister Nora who helped me first. She had faith in me. I figured I couldn't be too bad."

In 1969, Sister Nora left the hospital to take a position at the College of Saint Teresa. Roger Wells, 26 years old, became the new personnel director. To his shock, Roger learned that his predecessor worked 14-hour days and much of each weekend. Roger's story is part of a later chapter, but his remark about Sister Nora seems appropriate here: "Sister Nora might be a very small woman, but I knew I had big shoes to fill."

In the early 1950s, personnel faced the challenge of finding qualified persons to staff the large new hospital addition under construction. In 1939, just prior to the war, the Sisters developed a comprehensive building plan and implemented it with dispatch in the postwar period. Their objective was to provide Mayo with facilities for medical advances developed during World War II. Dave Leonard recalled the Sisters' response to Mayo's need for new facilities. "Mayo had the Sisters' complete trust. The Franciscans were not subservient; it was their choice. There was never any question about money—they went forward with whatever facilities were needed at the time."

Sister Domitilla chaired the building committee for the hospital's seven-story addition completed in 1956, named in her honor. As chair, she drew up a list of priority recommendations. Surprisingly, it was housekeeping, not new construction, that headed her list. "That the housekeeping department be organized under a qualified person who has demonstrated her ability to handle such an important assignment." The addition of 220 beds in the new building gave Saint Marys the potential of 1,000 beds, "the largest private hospital under one roof in the United States." Maintaining the cleanliness and good order of Saint Marys was an imperative.

Sister Lucas Chavez was appointed head housekeeper in 1951, a position she held until 1975. Small in stature like Sister Nora, Sister Lucas was another Franciscan with a focused mission and unbounded energy to see it accomplished. Unlike most Sisters who changed from the traditional habit to street dress in the 1960s, Sister Lucas always wore the full Franciscan habit. The habit framed a lovely face and sweet smile that endeared her to patients, employees, and Sisters alike. Sister Lucas seemed to personify the tribute Bishop Fitzgerald paid the Sisters at the dedication of the new addition: ". . . to the hundreds of hidden lives of prayer, sacrifice, and work that make this institution possible."

Sister Lucas came well pre-pared for her new assignment. Formerly supervisor of floor housekeepers, she and "her ladies," as she always called them, cared for the patient rooms, offices, class-rooms, and doctors' quarters. Sister Lucas stressed the importance of guarding patients against infection. Housekeepers learned how to

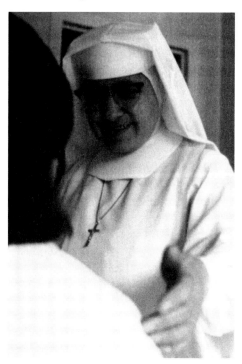

Sister Lucas Chavez served as head house-keeper from 1951 to 1975. (From Caring, Winter 1980, p 4. Rochester, MN: Saint Marys Hospital.)

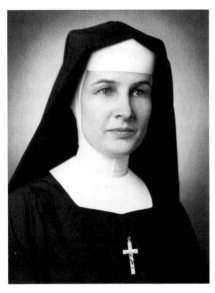

Sister Generose Gervais served in a variety of positions prior to her appointment as hospital Administrator. (From Saint Marys Hospital Archives.)

clean isolation rooms and how to manage and prevent infections.

Sister Lucas and Sister Generose Gervais, then assistant administrator, worked together to address the needs of the growing department. Sister Generose, a hands-on administrator who walked miles of Saint Mary's corridors each day, "knew every nook and cranny of the operation." Lifelong friends, the two Sisters were an excellent working team. After carefully studying each housekeeping position, they drew up a tentative job description and work schedule. Before approving the position, Sister Lucas first worked the schedule herself, "to be sure an average good worker had enough to do, but not too much."

"Lost and Found" was Sister Generose's responsibility and she asked Sister Lucas to help her. Sister Lucas handled patient claims, a charge that sometimes required the talents of a sleuth. Unclaimed items were sorted and packed in large, neatly labeled boxes. Before storing, all clothing items were cleaned and washed. "Lost and Found" held the boxes for about a year, then sent them to charity. Making the rounds of the building each day, Sister Lucas automatically picked up unattended items—to the dismay of one visitor. A pharmaceutical representative left his coat on a bench outside the pharmacy when he went inside to take an order. As he left, pharmacists heard him shout. "Hey! There's a nun running off with my coat!" Needless to say, he had no problem retrieving the item from Sister Lucas.

Sister Lucas headed a legion of Sisters and Franciscan novices assigned to clean the new Domitilla Building. As was the practice after all construction, Sisters did the final cleaning. Without benefit of air conditioning, they worked on the new addition over the summer of 1956. Franciscan novices came from the motherhouse during the day. At night Saint Marys Sisters helped mop, scrape, and clean "every inch of new space," as one of them recalled. "After a twelve-hour day, we went to the Domitilla building and worked from seven to ten. Then we'd go to the dining room and Sister Moira [Tighe] always had a big tray of delicious meat sandwiches."

Closely allied with housekeeping, the sewing room had a new supervisor in 1951, Sister Ellen Klooster, who held the position for 39 years. Sister Ellen and her capable workers had three areas of responsibility: the sewing room proper, the mending room, and the upholstery shop. In the sewing room, seamstresses made new articles, from draperies to surgical linens to supplies for pediatrics. In the mending room "not even the tiniest hole escaped the searching eyes of expert menders." Chairs came apart in the upholstery shop and springs were recast, frames glued, and cushions recovered.

Sister Ellen knew as much about sewing and fabrics as a mechanic knows about engines. She was also a remarkable organizer and kept a Kardex file with a card for every room in the hospital. Room 4-149, for example, had drapes that were 9 feet, 2 inches long with beige background and blue mums. The walls were beige and the chair an off-white upholstery. The cards, which recorded dates of installation, also gave a good idea of the wearability of fabric and the remodeling rotation.

Sister Ellen and her crew made draperies for all the windows in the new unit as they did for every window in the hospital. In addition, they meticulously repaired, cleaned, and refabricated the draperies. "With that kind of care," noted Sister Ellen, "our draperies lasted 15 to 20 years." "Time never dragged in the sewing room," she remembered, "I enjoyed my work

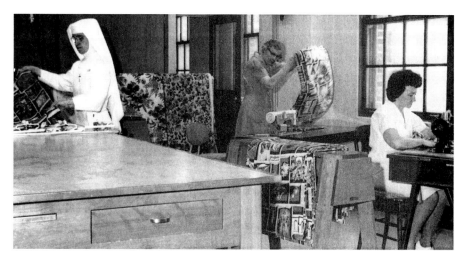

Sister Ellen Klooster, supervisor of the sewing room for 39 years, with her dedicated staff. "We were family for each other," said Sister Ellen. (From Saint Marys Hospital Archives.)

and was happy to challenge my skills and use the gifts I have for the good of Saint Marys. Above all, I didn't do it alone. I had wonderful, dedicated workers. We were family for each other."

The average person visiting Saint Marys had little knowledge of housekeeping or sewing room functions, beyond admiring the hospital's cleanliness and efficiency. Almost everyone, however, was vitally interested in the new clinical areas of physical medicine and rehabilitation and psychiatric services as well as the emergency room and intensive care unit. Sister Mary Brigh outlined these new areas in several public presentations. An entire floor of the new wing would provide rehabilitation for patients suffering from strokes and nerve or bone injuries, as well as polio patients. Noting the increased need for facilities to treat mentally ill patients, she described new facilities for psychiatric diagnosis and short-term treatment. She explained the reason for an expanded emergency room. "When this service was opened in 1942, it was thought it would be more than adequate. But in the ten years from 1942 to 1952, the number of admissions through the emergency room increased 420 percent. . .Fifty percent of all patients coming to Saint Marys enter through the back door—the emergency room. The new and greatly enlarged emergency service will be located at the front of the structure instead of the rear."

Built with a circular drive and space for clinical and office needs, the emergency room jutted out from the main structure. The design provided additional space for hospitalized patients on the floors above. A neurosurgery intensive care unit, not included in the original blueprints, had its origins in this design.

Intensive care units in the early 1950s were almost unknown. Government studies referred to ICUs as a division of "progressive patient care." Saint Marys Hospital was one the first hospitals to implement the concept. A 1958 *Hospital Progress* article authored by Sisters Mary Brigh and Amadeus Klein noted that the intensive care unit "was a natural outgrowth of successful experience with post-anesthesia recovery rooms in the operating room and delivery room suites. We believed that if the special equipment and services available for a short time in these areas could be extended to critically ill patients for a longer period, better patient care would result."

Sister Amadeus, a teacher who volunteered as nurse's aide during World War II, transferred to nursing in 1947. After earning a baccalaureate degree in nursing, she was appointed supervisor in neurology. Sister Amadeus later wrote about her early experiences in the unit. "In our 116-bed neurological and neurosurgical division, there were always a number of critically ill patients who needed almost constant observation. Checking of pulse, respiration, reflexes and responses at 15-minute intervals is a routine order for many of them . . . it was natural that we would think of this group of patients as the one for which an intensive care unit should be planned."

When Sister Amadeus saw the first blueprints of the new addition, she noted the sizable area that jutted out for the emergency room on the main floor. She proposed that neurology, located directly on the floor above, use this area for an intensive care unit to serve "the very sickest and the new postoperative patients who required more intensive nursing care." Sister Amadeus approached Sister Domitilla with the idea. After careful assessment of the rationale and supporting evidence, Sister Domitilla gave the project her full support. Sister Amadeus, with her nursing colleagues, developed recommendations for the architects' implementation.

In the summer of 1954, Sister Domitilla suffered a stroke shortly after she finished teaching a science class to LPN students. Sister Sharon Hooley recalled the incident well, "I had just gotten off the elevator when I saw Sister Mary Brigh gently cradling Sister Domitilla as they waited for staff to bring a gurney." After 7 months of critical illness, Sister Domitilla died February 17, 1955. She was 65 years old. Later that year, Sister Mary Brigh announced that the new addition would be named for Sister Domitilla. "Gifted by God with a clarity of vision that was akin to genius," she "exercised an influence, second to none, in the growth and development of the hospital and schools of nursing." Not one of the pioneer Sisters, she had the more exacting task of "re-organizing, strengthening, and expanding the service of the early days so that nothing that was good in the past might be lost and nothing of value in the present and future might be overlooked or rejected."

Sister Domitilla at the same time that she chaired the hospital building committee, also chaired the building committee for the new Franciscan motherhouse. "She had an unusual appreciation of beauty in structure and natural materials," commented Sister Mary Brigh. "Both of these buildings will forever bear traces of her careful planning and sure instinct for what is right in design."

Since the early 1930s, Sister Domitilla was a trusted advisor for two major superiors, Mother Aquinas Norton and her successor, Mother Alcuin McCarthy. During Mother Alcuin's administration (1946-1958), unprecedented numbers of young women joined the congregation. The number of new Sisters created a space problem for the small motherhouse downtown, which had no adjoining land for expansion. The Franciscans needed a larger structure and a new location. Within months of election, Mother Alcuin addressed the issue with her council and appointed a building committee under Sister Domitilla.

Following their practice of consulting with Mayo leaders about hospital issues, Franciscans approached Harry Harwick for advice about property for the new motherhouse. With Harwick's assistance, they purchased prime land in northwest Rochester, 138 acres situated on a bluff overlooking the city.

A simple ceremony marked the laying of the cornerstone on July 10, 1953. Two years later, Bishop Fitzgerald dedicated the new motherhouse on October 4, 1955, the congregation's 75th anniversary. Italian romanesque in architecture, the new motherhouse resembled the Basilica of St. Francis in Assisi in color, stone, and red tile roofing. Like the basilica, Assisi Heights sat on a hilltop looking down on a rolling green valley. The large congregational center housed several buildings under one roof: administrative offices, congregational novitiate, retirement and health care center, educational facilities, and a retreat center for laity.

The property, later known as Assisi Heights, consisted of the homestead of a local farmer and the estate of Louis B. Wilson, M.D. The Wilson property held particular significance for the hospital Sisters. Dr. Wilson came to Mayo in 1905. The Clinic's first pathologist, he developed the fresh frozen tissue method for pathological diagnosis in surgery. Dr. Wilson, whose laboratory was near the operating rooms at Saint Marys, worked closely with Sister

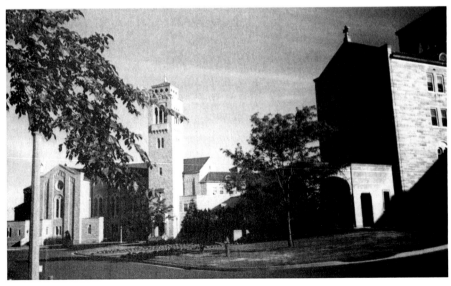

Assisi Heights, motherhouse of the Sisters of Saint Francis, was dedicated on October 4, 1955, the congregation's 75th anniversary. (Courtesy of Sister Bernadine Jax.)

Joseph and the founding Franciscans. To the Sisters, Dr. Wilson was not only a gifted scientist, but also a dear friend and trusted colleague.

Born and raised in the farmlands of Pennsylvania, Dr. Wilson had an avid interest in horticulture. After purchasing the property that would become Assisi Heights, Dr. Wilson planted his first orchard in 1925. Until his death in 1943, he worked on the orchard with horticulturists from the University of Minnesota. In 1949, the year of the Sisters' purchase, Dr. Wilson's apple orchard had grown to 25 acres. The 1,375 apple trees represented more than 40 varieties of apples, among them, several new varieties developed by Dr. Wilson and his university colleagues.

Dr. Wilson spoke eloquently about the Sisters and Saint Marys Hospital. "Saint Marys is like no other hospital; its tradition is real mercy and kindness. These Sisters are not noted for their business management, though it is marvelous, nor for their courage in erecting great buildings, but for their real, womanly kindness. Their human interest in the individual patient has always made Saint Marys more a home than a hospital. That is what we physicians will always think of as the outstanding trait of the Sisters." Dr. Wilson would have been pleased that his orchard provided bountiful fruit for the Sisters and not surprised that they shared their harvest with Saint Marys Hospital patients and staff.

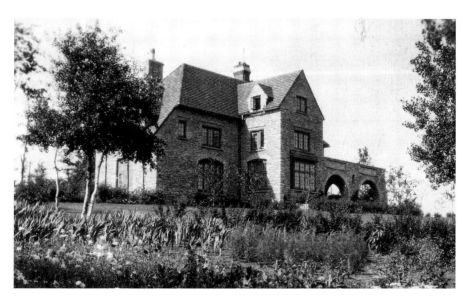

Walnut Hill farm, the home of Louis B. Wilson, M.D., later became part of Assisi Heights. (From Nelson C: Mayo and the Potato King. Mayo Today 1993 Oct;4 no. 8:20.)

ENDNOTES

Page 115   *A Century of Caring: 1889-1989.* Rochester, MN: Saint Marys Hospital, 1988, pp 89-90.

Johnson V: *Mayo Clinic: Its Growth and Progress.* Bloomington, MN: Voyageur Press, 1984, p 78.

Hockema M: *The Franciscan Five.* p 31 (unpublished paper).

Dr. W. Eugene Mayberry's remarks at the dedication of the Mary Brigh Building, September 30, 1980.

Saint Marys Hospital News Bulletin Vol. 30, Special Issue, October 1971, p 5.

Walle P: Sister Mary Brigh: A Pioneer in Medical Services. *Rochester Post-Bulletin* September 23, 1971, p 12.

Page 116   Hockema (pp 31-32).

Roosevelt University—History of Chicago: *History of Chicago From Trading Post to Metropolis.* Module 3, chapter 2, p 1. [cited 2006 February 2]. Available from: http://www.encyclopedia.chicagohistory.org/pages/542.html. pp 1-2.

Page 117   It Is Always Only Today. *Saint Marys Hospital News Bulletin* October 1971, p 4.

Rochester Post-Bulletin March 21, 1952, p 8.

Page 118   Saint Marys Personnel Department. *Saint Marys Hospital News Bulletin* November 1945, p 5.

Pages 118-119 Interview with Margaret Hermann, August 8, 2005.

Page 119   Interview with Sister Valerie Olson, September 22, 2005.

Interview with Anne Purrington, February 20, 2006.

Interview with Sister Neal Logan, September 21, 2005.

Pages 119-120 Interview with Sister Fidelis Logan, July 26, 2005.

Page 120 Interview with Ray Island, February 22, 2006.

Interview with Roger Wells, February 9, 2006.

Pages 120-121 Interview with David A. Leonard, July 18, 2003.

Saint Marys Hospital Archives. Sister Domitilla papers.

Page 122 *The Courier* **October 4, 1956, p 1.**

Interview with Sister Generose Gervais, February 22, 2005 and March 31, 2006.

Saint Marys Hospital News Bulletin **November 1965, p 5.**

Page 123 Interview with Sister Ellen Klooster, September 2, 2006.

Saint Marys Hospital News Bulletin **April 1968, p 5.**

Page 124 **Sister Ellen Klooster.** *Caring* **Summer 1989, p 8.**

Seven Story Unit Will Replace Most of Oldest Building: Saint Marys Plans Are Disclosed. *Rochester Post-Bulletin* **October 23, 1953, p 1.**

Sister Mary Brigh, Sister Mary Amadeus: Intensive Care: Effective Care. Reprinted from *Hospital Progress* **December 1958.**

Page 125 **Klein, Sister Amadeus:** *Neurological and Neurosurgical Nursing, Saint Marys Hospital, Rochester, Minnesota: 1947-1960.* **pp 1-6 (unpublished paper).**

Saint Marys Hospital News Bulletin **December 1955, p 3.**

Interview with Sister Sharon Hooley (Patricia Hooley), March 7, 2005.

Saint Marys Hospital News Bulletin **March 1955, p 1.**

Page 126 **Franciscan Congregational Council Minutes. February 1, 1949; May 4, 1949; July 5, 1949.**

Franciscan Sisters Soon to Build New Motherhouse, Novitiate Here. *Rochester Post-Bulletin* **November 28, 1949.**

City Seated on a Hill. *The Courier Motherhouse Dedication Supplement* October 16, 1955.

Page 127   *A Franciscan Symphony of Courage & Creativity*. Rochester, MN: Assisi Heights and Saint Marys Hospital Archives, pp 15-16.

Nelson CW: *Mayo Roots: Profiling the Origins of Mayo Clinic*. Rochester, MN: Mayo Historical Unit, Mayo Foundation, 1990, pp 238-239, 304-305.

Saint Marys Hospital Annals, 1922.

CHAPTER 7

Advancing Patient Care

O n a fall afternoon, bright with sunshine and autumn colors, 800 guests strolled across the Saint Marys campus. It was September 30, 1956—the hospital's 67th anniversary and dedication day for the Domitilla wing. Ceremonies began in chapel with a solemn blessing followed by a program in the auditorium. J. Minot Stickney, M.D., presided. Like most of the guests, Dr. Stickney was a colleague of the Franciscans. His opening remarks recalled the legacy of the pioneer Sisters. Even the numbers, he said, told a dramatic story. On this site in 1889, an unknown hospital opened with 27 beds. Sixty-seven years later, now almost 1,000 beds, Saint Marys was acclaimed across the world. "The Sisters of Saint Francis," he declared, "have a right to be proud on this occasion."

After his opening remarks, Dr. Stickney introduced the main speaker, internationally known psychiatrist Francis J. Braceland, M.D., president of the American Psychiatric Society. Formerly a member of the Mayo staff, Dr. Braceland distinguished himself as the first chair of the psychiatry department. Arriving in 1946, he led the rapidly growing section until his departure in 1951 to head the Institute for Living in Hartford, Connecticut. Dr. Braceland helped overcome the stigma of psychiatry present at Mayo at that time. His commitment to the medical model immediately recommended him to Clinic colleagues. A "will of steel" and sense of humor also served him well. "He was a genius," said one peer, "who made psychiatry happen at the Mayo Clinic."

A devout Catholic, Dr. Braceland viewed psychiatry as a spiritual journey. According to a colleague, Maurice J. Martin, M.D., "psychiatry was part of

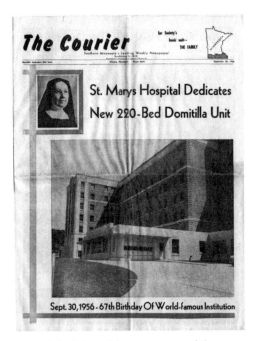

The Courier

Southern Minnesota's Leading Weekly Newspaper

St. Marys Hospital Dedicates New 220-Bed Domitilla Unit

Sept. 30, 1956 - 67th Birthday Of World-famous Institution

A special edition of the newspaper of the Diocese of Winona proclaimed the opening of the Domitilla Unit. (From The Courier. Winona, MN: Diocese of Winona. Used with permission.)

his religion." Born of modest means, his teachers, the Christian Brothers, encouraged him to go into medicine. During his studies, Braceland "crossed paths with others who would influence the development of psychiatry, not only in Rochester, but the nation." Howard P. Rome, M.D., who would later join him at Mayo, was among them. At the onset of World War II, both men enlisted in the Navy and received their commissions. Dr. Braceland persuaded the Navy Surgeon General to develop a neuropsychiatry branch, which he headed. "There were 8 psychiatrists in the Navy," writes M. J. Martin, "and 800 [sic] when the war was over."

Braceland's presentation at Saint Marys that day focused on a new approach to patient care, the interrelationship of the patient's body, mind, and spirit. "The patient is the center of the stage in the medical profession," he told his audience. "We need to integrate the latest advances of the physical and psychological fields with the spiritual. All three areas contribute to the whole of the patient."

Dr. Braceland paid tribute to the Sisters with high praise for the hospital's "spiritual atmosphere." He also pointed out that Saint Marys was one of the first general hospitals to admit mental patients. As noted earlier, Franciscan efforts to establish psychiatric services began in 1922, when Sister Joseph requested a psychiatric floor in the new surgery pavilion. The Sisters believed a psychiatric unit in a general hospital would promote early treatment and lessen the likelihood of long-term psychiatric care for many patients. At the time, psychiatry was not generally accepted as a medical specialty and her request was declined. In the opinion of Mayo leaders, psychiatric patients were not appropriate in a general hospital. In 1935, when Sister Domitilla proposed a psychiatric unit, Mayo colleagues again declined the request for the same reason. Undaunted, she sent two gifted Franciscans, Sisters Julié Erne and Helen Hayes, for advanced studies in psychiatric nursing. Attending the Catholic University of America, they had the good fortune to do their clinical work at St. Elizabeth's in Washington, D.C., a premier psychiatric hospital. Upon their return to Saint Marys, the Sisters incorporated treatment techniques gleaned from this experience.

During the 1940s, attitudes about psychiatric patients began to change. The neurology section, which treated an increasing number of psychiatric patients, made note of this in annual reports. "The management of psychiatric services continues to be a problem. It can only be improved by the provision of a special unit or room equipped for this purpose . . . The Sisters, especially Sister Domitilla [DuRocher], have come to our rescue by offering suitable quarters and trained nursing personnel for our psychiatric patients. We are indeed grateful for this offer of help." Concurrently, Mayo physicians returning from active service in World War II "recognized the enormity of the problem with thousands of service personnel either discharged or rejected from active duty because of psychiatric disorders."

It was in response to this new dynamic that the Board of Governors took several initiatives in 1946. The Section of Neurology became the Department of Neurology and Psychiatry, with Dr. Braceland head of the psychiatric section. In addition, Saint Marys Hospital established a 22-bed psychiatric unit with Sister Julié as nursing supervisor.

Treating the patient as a whole person—body, mind, and spirit—had important implications for nursing. Sister Domitilla had anticipated this development when she sent Sisters Julié and Helen (Sister Immaculata) for degrees in psychiatric nursing. Significantly, before retiring as hospital administrator, she appointed Sister Julié director of the school of nursing. Within the hospital's organizational structure, the appointment carried broad authority and influence. Sister Julié not only headed the school of nursing but also directed nursing service throughout Saint Marys.

In her new position, Sister Julié spoke to Rochester's Rotary Club about the changes in nursing. "Previously," she explained, "nursing emphasis was placed on *the diseased organ*, not on *the patient with a disease*." The new approach "points to an appreciation of the patient as a total personality." To care for the patient as a total person, body, mind, and spirit, "the nurse must understand the interrelationship of these factors and base her nursing approach on them."

With Sister Julié's appointment as nursing director, Sister Helen Hayes became nursing supervisor for psychiatry. Highly capable, with excellent interpersonal skills, Sister Helen brought her vision of psychiatric care to Saint Marys Hospital. As hospital administrator, Sister Mary Brigh Cassidy supported the service but kept her distance from its operation. Confident of Sister Helen's abilities, she delegated operational responsibilities to her. Almost single-handedly, Sister Helen created a hospital service for the new Mayo specialty. In that capacity, she worked closely with Dr. Braceland until he left Mayo. Subsequently, she worked with the able group of psychiatrists Dr. Braceland brought to Mayo, perhaps most notably Dr. Howard Rome, who succeeded him as section head.

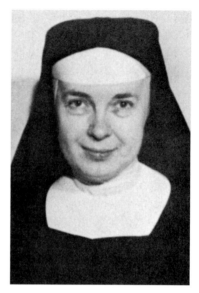

Sister Julié Erne not only headed Saint Marys School of Nursing but also directed nursing service throughout the hospital. (From Saint Marys Archives.)

An acclaimed teacher, Sister Helen not only directed the unit but also taught psychiatry to students in Saint Marys School of Nursing and the College of Saint Teresa's nursing program. Resident physicians in psychiatry also gained from her instruction. "Sister Helen," noted Dr. Martin, "taught many of us a good deal about patient care."

"Helen was the heart of the department," observed Marjorie Habenicht Overby (Sister Joris), who worked with Sister Helen in the 1960s. "She was the central figure who ran the department and related to administration, Mayo psychiatry, and the nursing schools." Psychiatry was Sister Mary Lynch's (Sister Mercy) first assignment at Saint Marys in 1956. "I was fortunate to get the assignment. I had trained as a nurse in a psychiatric hospital before I entered the convent. This background was probably the reason Sister Helen asked me to serve in psychiatry; she was very selective about staff, including Sisters. Helen was very helpful—she always had time for you. I enjoyed my years in psychiatry very much and worked with excellent residents like Dr. Bob Morse [Robert M. Morse, M.D.]."

Later on, Sister Helen would make an important contribution to other areas of Saint Marys, notably chaplaincy. Her dedication to psychiatry, however, left a lasting legacy. After her death, the department paid her tribute by dedicating "The Helen Hayes Conference Room" to her memory.

Emergency medicine also came to the fore during these years. Though minimally involved with psychiatry, Sister Mary Brigh's writings and personal interactions attest to her involvement with emergency room services. In a hospital publication, she traced the development of the department. Saint Marys first emergency room opened in the Francis building. "In its first full year of service, 1942," said Sister Mary Brigh, "it cared for 2,764 patients. It took awhile for people to get used to the idea of going to the hospital instead of staying home and hurting . . . But, before long, our Emergency Room was filled to overflowing. Emergency care was becoming an established part of hospital practice." In 1956, more than 7,000 patients visited the emergency room, necessitating a new and significantly enlarged facility in the Domitilla building.

"The emergency room," declared Pat Hooley (Sister Sharon), "was the best assignment I had in 50 years of nursing. I was supervisor from 1957 to 1965 and still remember what Sister Mary Brigh told me when I got the assignment, 'The Emergency Room and Admissions have the most important jobs in the hospital,' she said, 'you are the ones who make the first impression on patients. I expect that impression to be a good one.'"

"We thrived on challenges in the ER, internal and external. During my time, IBM opened a large plant in Rochester and the demand for ER services soared. The Cuban Missile Crisis brought new emphasis on preparedness. Under the direction of Jack Ivins, M.D., a noted surgeon, we conducted mock emergency drills in the city and around the state using simulated injuries and fake wounds. Dedicated physicians like Dr. Ed Henderson [Edward

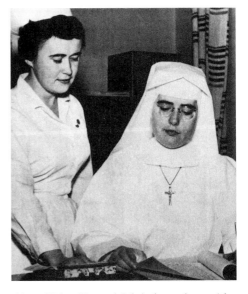

Sister Helen Hayes (right) shown here with Miss Jean Hennessey (left), directed the psychiatry unit and taught psychiatry to students in Saint Marys School of Nursing and the College of Saint Teresa's nursing program. (From Assisi Heights Archives.)

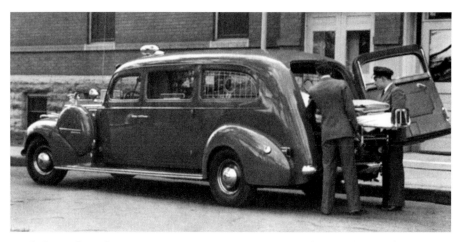

Ambulances brought many patients to Saint Marys Hospital as the demand for emergency care soared. (From A Century of Caring: 1889-1989. Rochester, MN: Saint Marys Hospital, 1988, p 65.)

D. Henderson, M.D.] and Dr. Tony Bianco [Anthony J. Bianco, Jr., M.D.] taught me a great deal. I could still take lessons in spiritual care from Alice Haldorson, an outstanding nurse, who succeeded me as ER supervisor."

Charlotte "Char" Carey worked in the emergency room as a student nurse in 1965. "It was the most fun I ever had—no day was the same. After graduation, I went to the ER and stayed 23 years, about half the time as head nurse. I liked the challenge of thinking on my feet. We had no permanent medical staff; physician consultation was on-call only. Residents rotated through the ER and nurses, for all purposes, trained them. Several staff physicians helped us out on their own time, among them, Richard Bryan [Richard S. Bryan, M.D.], orthopedics, Douglas McGill [Douglas B. McGill, M.D.], gastroenterology, and Tony Bianco, orthopedic surgery. After Vietnam, physicians came back to Mayo with experience in emergency medicine; during the seventies, staff physicians took an active leadership role in the ER with residents and staff."

"I liked every part of the job," Char continued, "especially making a difference for patients. A patient I'll always remember was an 18-year-old girl who was raped and didn't want her parents to know. While a nursing colleague covered for me, I spent time with the young girl. Eventually, friends came to get her. Before leaving, she told me, 'I just hope I can help someone like you helped me today.' For me, that's the difference nursing can make."

In the ER and throughout the hospital, the polio epidemics of the 1940s and 1950s left indelible memories. Marlene Staley served as staff nurse in the first emergency room. Ambulances arrived daily with new patients. Parents crowded outside the emergency room while their children received spinal taps to confirm the diagnosis. "There were tense moments waiting for that first drop of spinal fluid," recalled Marlene. "I can vividly remember the anxiety of patients with fevers, stiff necks, or muscle weakness." Nursing supervisor, Sister Regina Buskowiak (Sister Raymond), remembers a gentleman who came to the emergency room. "He walked in the door, but by the time we gave him a spinal tap, he could no longer walk. The disease progressed that quickly!" Later, as supervisor in Physical Medicine and Rehabilitation from 1955 to 1962, Sister Regina cared for polio patients she first met in the emergency room.

The most seriously ill patients were placed in iron lungs, the large cylindrical machines that rhythmically simulate the paralyzed breathing muscles that no longer contracted involuntarily. Other patients, many of whom could not move their arms or legs, went to the isolation ward. At the

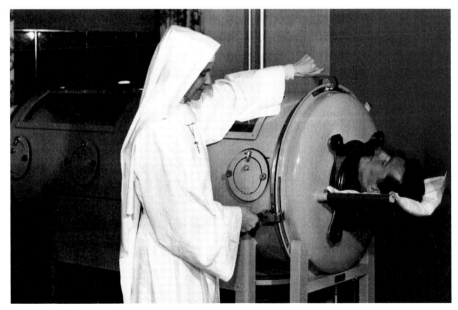

As supervisor in the Department of Physical Medicine and Rehabilitation, Sister Regina Buskowiak oversaw the care of many patients stricken with polio. Here, she cares for a patient in an iron lung. (From A Century of Caring: 1889-1989. Rochester, MN: Saint Marys Hospital, 1988, p 64.)

height of the epidemics, cots were placed in the halls, 2 or 3 feet apart, to accommodate all the patients.

The polio years abound with stories of patients and caregivers, heart-rending tales of heroism, self-sacrifice, and sometimes, just good luck. Dr. Hal Wente [Harold A. Wente, M.D.], told such a story. "I had never done a tracheotomy, but I started one at Saint Marys Hospital in 1952. It was a Sunday morning. My wife Elaine had just gotten the children dressed for Mass when I received a call from a patient whose 10-year-old son was having trouble breathing. I left my family standing in front of our house and drove to a farm south of Rochester. I found the child in acute respiratory distress from bulbar polio. The mother was alone in the house except for a small infant and another child. I carried the boy to the car, put him in the front seat with me, and drove at great speed to Saint Marys.

When I arrived at the ER, only the Sister in charge was present. Barely alive, my patient stopped breathing when I placed him on the table. I told Sister, 'Get a surgeon, he'll need a tracheotomy.' She said, 'I'll call one, but he won't get here in time. Here's a scalpel.' I gulped hard and made a vertical incision in the boy's neck and started to make a horizontal opening into the trachea. Just then, a good friend, Bernie Spencer [Bernard Spencer, M.D.],

arrived on the scene. He made the opening and I put the scalpel handle into the incision. The patient coughed and began breathing normally. I still see the boy's mother and father around town. I see the boy less frequently, but always recognize him by the ugly vertical scar on his neck."

The stories of Mayo employees C. Dale Rustad (below) and Sandy Hanson, both patients at Saint Marys, attest to polio's far-reaching impact. "I was 8 years old, a third grader, when I contracted polio in 1948. In September and October of 1948, 10 children in our community southeast of Rochester came down with polio. In one case, 3 in one family and 2 brothers in another family died of polio. They were friends of mine; we rode the school bus together. School closed for 3 weeks and everything in town

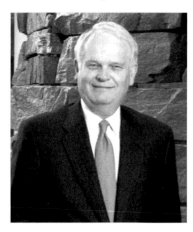

C. Dale Rustad recovered from polio at Saint Marys when he was 8 years old. Dale recently celebrated 45 years of service at Mayo. (From Mayo Magazine, Autumn 2004, p 8. Rochester, MN: Mayo Foundation for Medical Education and Research.)

was cancelled, football games and all public events. The city sprayed the streets and alleys with DDT. We didn't have another case of polio.

"I developed muscular pain and a severe headache," Dale recalled. "My parents took me to a doctor in nearby Lanesboro, because he sent all his patients to Saint Marys. We drove to Rochester in the family car and arrived late that evening. I'll never forget it. From the emergency room, I went to the isolation ward with 10 other boys and stayed 2 weeks. We couldn't see anyone, but my mother wrote wonderful letters and slipped them under the door. From the isolation ward, I went to rehabilitation for therapy that included hot packs and the whirlpool. My condition improved. I was able to go home in about 2 months and returned for outpatient therapy 60 times. Fortunately, not long before I came down with the disease, my parents had taken polio insurance which covered all the expenses.

"The love and compassion I received from the physicians, the Sisters of Saint Francis, and the entire staff, was overwhelming to me, even as a child," said Dale. "It also meant a great deal to my parents. We aren't Catholic, but religious denominations blur at such times. Our visits to Saint Marys beautiful chapel gave us comfort and strength. I'll never forget the care and concern of the Sisters, and to this day feel a special bond with them."

Recently, Dale celebrated 45 years of service at Mayo. "Little did I know that my professional career would bring me back to the Mayo Clinic. In every position I've held—from managing the Foundation House to my current role in the Department of Development—I've been able to pass along the Mayo values I experienced as a child in Saint Marys Hospital."

Sandy Hanson, a Mayo telephone operator for 36 years, contracted polio in 1952. At 11 months old, she was paralyzed in both legs and her right arm. Sandy tells her own story: "The doctors at Saint Marys told my parents I wouldn't be able to go home for awhile—I didn't leave the hospital for

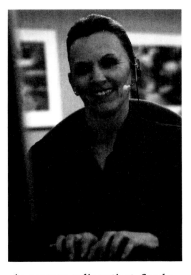

As a young polio patient, Sandy Hanson dreamed of someday "helping people in the hospital." Today she works in the telephone office at Saint Marys Hospital, assisting patients, family members, and staff. (From Vision in Action. This Week at Mayo Clinic, 2005 April 29;15:3.)

a year, and then only for short periods. My sister and brother couldn't come to visit me. My Grandma would take me out on the balcony and hold me up so they could see me. I can still see them sitting on the lawn, looking up and waving at me."

"I remember going to therapy day after day," Sandy recalled, "all day long, stopping long enough for lunch and going again till suppertime. I lay under the heat lamps that were so hot I wanted to scream and went into the whirlpool for hours at a time. At night in bed, I'd listen for my mother's footsteps—I could always tell them. Every night I'd hear the Sisters coming down the hall in their swishing habits, their rosaries made a little click. I knew I'd better try to go to sleep before they came to my room! My mom and dad and the hospital staff kept me going with their love and encouragement. By the time I was three, I walked alone with crutches, but I still had a long way to go."

"By the time I was 16, I'd had 12 surgeries, followed by hospitalization and therapy. Everyone at Saint Marys treated me like family, the doctors, the Sisters, all the staff. Because of the way I was treated, I was never afraid to come back to the hospital for more surgery. My last surgery was a big one. I was in a body cast for several months. I'll never forget Sister Ruth Peterson in orthopedics. Every day, she took time to visit and encourage me. I remember Sister JoAnne Lawson too, she told me wonderful stories. It was all worth it, now only my left leg is paralyzed and I can walk with a brace."

"I saw my doctors every 3 months for many years. They were so good to me, especially Dr. Janes [Joseph M. Janes, M.D.] and Dr. Henderson [Edward D. Henderson, M.D.]. Dr. Henderson once asked me what I wanted to be when I grew up; I was 5 or 6 at the time. I told him I wanted to be just like him—help people in the hospital. During high school, when I passed the hospital telephone office, I'd think, 'That would be a good place to work.' I applied and got the job. I didn't become a doctor or a nurse, but I'm helping people every day on the telephone at Saint Marys. I can feel their pain, their worries, and their fears. I've been down that road. If I make patients, family members, or staff feel a little better on the phone, then I've done what I set out to do. I have the best job I could have at Mayo."

With the development of the Salk vaccine in 1955, the polio epidemics ended. Vaccine inoculations virtually eliminated the disease. When the new Domitilla building opened in 1956, the physical medicine and rehabilitation space planned for polio patients became available for patients suffering from other physical symptoms, such as strokes and bone and nerve injuries.

"The very early history of the Department of Physical Medicine and Rehabilitation (PM&R) at Mayo Clinic," writes Joachim L. Opitz, M.D., "started in the Department of Orthopedic Surgery soon after its inception in 1912. The founder of the Department of Orthopedic Surgery and of its 'Physiotherapy' was Melvin S. Henderson, M.D. In 1924, a second physical therapy department, the Diathermy Department (later called the 'Electrotherapy Department') was established by Arthur U. Desjardins, M.D., as part of the Department of Therapeutic Radiology. These 2 individual therapy departments coexisted at the Clinic from 1924 to 1935."

In the early 1930s, Mayo recognized the value of combining the two programs and looked outward for leadership. Then in its formative stage, physical medicine had a remarkable proponent in Frank H. Krusen, M.D., of Temple University. Krusen, after undergoing treatment for tuberculosis, made physical medicine his career and established a physical therapy program at Temple. Impressed by Krusen's dynamic leadership, Dr. Henderson invited him to join Mayo in 1935.

Within a year, Dr. Krusen combined the root programs into the Section of Physical Therapy and established the first physical medicine residency program. On the national scene, he proposed the term "physiatrist" to identify the physician specializing in physical medicine. Over the next decade, Krusen helped establish physical medicine and rehabilitation as a medical specialty.

Reviewing the department's history, Mayo physiatrist, Robert W. DePompolo, M.D., observed, "World War II significantly broadened the focus of physical medicine. Physiatrists recognized that veterans of World War I deteriorated rapidly without rehabilitation. They set new treatment goals." "For the first time," Dr. DePompolo continued, "physical medicine took a comprehensive view of injured veterans and treated them holistically. Under Dr. Krusen, the department added exercise modality and blended rehabilitation. Social and spiritual components were vital for rehabilitation, as was vocational counseling. Wounded veterans of World War II overwhelmingly responded to rehabilitation and went on to lead productive lives."

During World War II, philanthropist and physical medicine proponent Bernard Baruch established the "Baruch Committee" and appointed Dr. Krusen executive director. According to Mayo physiatrist Joachim L. Opitz, M.D., the committee had two immediate goals: "to identify the most urgent financial needs of the fledgling specialty of physical medicine and address them with research and training grants." The Baruch Committee recommended PM&R teaching and research centers in universities and medical centers along

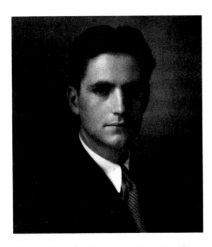

When Earl C. Elkins, M.D., joined the medical staff in 1939, he worked with patients hospitalized with major physical impairments such as spinal cord injuries and strokes. (From Opitz JL, DePompolo RW. History of the Mayo Clinic Department of Physical Medicine and Rehabilitation, 1911-2002. Rochester, MN: Mayo Foundation for Medical Education and Research, 2005, p 29.)

with fellowships and residencies, and promotion of PM&R in medical schools. In addition, they advocated wartime and post-war physician rehabilitation training and the development of an American Board of Physical Medicine and Rehabilitation.

The first resident trained in Mayo's PM&R program, Earl C. Elkins, M.D., became the second physiatrist on the Mayo staff in 1939. Dr. Elkins complemented Dr. Krusen in his interests and treatment specialties. While Dr. Krusen concentrated on outpatients in the Mayo building downtown, Dr. Elkins worked with hospitalized patients at Saint Marys Hospital, where major physical impairments, such as spinal cord injuries and strokes, were his central focus.

The Sisters at Saint Marys recognized the importance of Dr. Elkins' work and opened a 17-bed rehabilitation unit in 1947. When he heard about the new unit, Dr. Krusen wrote in his diary. "Earl Elkins came in right after lunch to tell me that we would have a 17-bed Physical Medicine unit at Saint Marys and I am delighted with this arrangement . . . [We can] develop a well-coordinated rehabilitation program at Saint Marys Hospital."

The achievements of Dr. Elkins and his team increased demand for services at Saint Marys. In response, the building committee provided an entire floor for the department in the Domitilla wing, more than twice the previous area. Nursing supervisor Sister Regina Buskowiak (Sister Raymond) helped the section move to their new quarters. Recalling her years in rehabilitation, Sister Regina spoke of Dr. Elkins, "I especially appreciated Dr. Elkins' skills and dedication in treating young people. We had many of them, accident victims and polio patients."

Sister Regina also praised the nursing staff: "Their duties were heavy, not only physically with paralyzed patients, but also psychologically. Immediately after an accident, patients were grateful to be alive. It wasn't long, however, before many suffered serious depression as they faced profound lifetime limitations. Some patients also lost spouses who were unable to live with the new reality. We had patients who could only move one finger to work the electric wheel chair." Sister Germaine Hullerman (Sister Roxanne) served as a staff nurse in rehabilitation from 1980 to 1992. She worked tirelessly to help patients learn to help themselves. "When our patients became able to take care of themselves," she recalled, "I truly rejoiced."

Franciscans at Saint Marys, whether nurses or not, had great interest in PM&R patients and staff. The department's location, adjacent to the convent and chapel, provided regular contact. Claire E. Bender, M.D., whose Mayo career began as a student in physical therapy, was unacquainted with Sisters before coming to Saint Marys. "The Sisters' dedication and values impressed me from the time I came to the medical center. I remember watching Sisters go in and out of chapel several times a day. I can still see one of them, an older Sister in full habit, who was visually impaired. She walked along the edge of the corridor, close to the wall as she went from chapel to work in the kitchen. Her quiet dedication made a lasting impression."

Dr. Bender, who went on to study medicine and specialize in radiology at Mayo, became a staff physician and member of the Board of Governors. Looking back, Dr. Bender spoke about her first years in PM&R. "The opportunity to work with a highly dedicated staff was of great value to me as a young person. It set the stage for my service at Mayo."

In the late 1940s, plans for the Domitilla building went forward on Saint Marys' campus and other changes unfolded downtown. The Kahler Corporation, that owned and operated downtown hospitals in its hotel/hospital facilities, reluctantly confronted "getting out of the hospital business." An integral part of Mayo's medical presence in Rochester, the impressive history of the Kahler hospitals began in 1906. By 1921, Kahler hospitals contained 1,000 patient beds in 6 dowtown locations. In addition, the Kahler School of Nursing held high national standing among training schools.

Mayo communications consultant William "Bill" Holmes described the corporation's difficult situation. "Kahler Corporation, by definition, was designed to be a profit-making organization . . . increasingly it faced more obstacles, taxes and more taxes." Changing tax laws, a major burden on for-profit hospitals, depleted Kahler hospital earnings by more than 75 percent. In 1947, when Kahler executive Roy Watson, Sr., advised Mayo of another increase in hospital rates, he noted, "Operations are on a very dangerous margin."

Downtown hospitals required new direction and management; Mayo began a quiet search for a provider. In 1953, Mayo informed the Kahler Corporation that the Methodist Board of Hospitals and Homes had "expressed an interest in taking over the downtown hospital function." The next year, Kahler and the Methodists settled the transfer of physical assets and the Kahler School of Nursing.

"Now all that had to be done," Holmes noted wryly, "was for the Methodists to bring about a medical/economic miracle." Providentially, a wide variety of individuals and groups joined forces to assist them. Several Mayo physicians spearheaded the effort; Samuel F. Haines, M.D., chair of Mayo's Board of Governors from 1947 to 1955, and Oliver H. Beahrs, M.D., whose medical center study on patient care made a strong impact on the new hospital were among the leaders. Outstanding contributions also came from 2 administrators, Gerald M. Needham, Ph.D., president of the new hospital's governing board, and Harold C. Mickey, first administrator and executive director.

Two Rochester newcomers also played critical roles, Harry A. Blackmun and Ralph Jester. Blackmun, then Mayo's legal counsel, later Associate Justice of the U.S. Supreme Court, came to Rochester in 1950. Two years later, businessman Ralph Jester made his first trip to Rochester from Des Moines, Iowa, "to look into the possibility of a church-related hospital." A member of the Board of Hospitals and Homes of the Methodist Church, Jester visited church-supported hospitals across the country. He met with Dr. Haines and Mayo colleagues, administrators from Saint Marys Hospital, and Kahler executives. "I am greatly enthused over the possibilities," Jester wrote Harry Blackmun. "In my judgment the Methodists have never had so challenging an opportunity."

Jester later recalled, "We didn't have a dime to start with." In a fund-raising campaign, he approached Iowa colleagues who responded generously. Iowans set the example, and Rochester donors followed with significant support. Jester's importance, however, went well beyond fund-raising. "He saw, perhaps before anyone in Rochester," wrote Holmes, "precisely where the new hospital must be located to interact more effectively with growing patient care/education/research efforts." Jester's vision persisted over the difficult decade that Methodist Hospital funded temporary "patch and paint improvements" of existing Kahler units. His leadership was largely responsible for creating "from dream to architectural concept to construction, a genuinely new entity, all in one grand sweep." In large part, Jester's vision

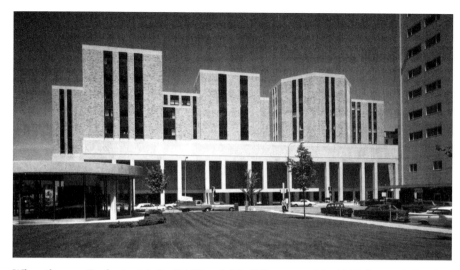

When the new Rochester Methodist Hospital building opened in 1966, it consolidated all the downtown hospital functions in one site. (From Mayo Clinic Archives.)

became a reality in 1966 at the dedication of the 800-bed facility with its radical new hospital design. Furthermore, Methodist Hospital was dedicated on a site that included a street vacated by the city to accommodate the desire for a key location close to the Clinic.

Reflecting on Jester's contribution to Rochester Methodist Hospital (RMH), Harry Blackmun observed, "He was, quite simply, of inestimable value." Interestingly, Blackmun's friends and colleagues would say the same of him. Harry Blackmun, a prominent lay Methodist, was deeply committed to a Methodist hospital in Rochester. Impressed with the Methodist Hospital System before he came to Rochester, Blackmun believed the hospital held great promise for the medical center. "If we can just get it off the ground," he said, "it has to work, it has to be good!"

Visiting with Harry Blackmun, Bill Holmes asked him to name a few persons who helped make Rochester Methodist Hospital a reality. Of the Mayo group, he noted Charles W. Mayo, M.D. (Dr. Chuck), Dr. Haines, and Mr. Harry Harwick. At the Kahler Corporation, "Roy Watson, senior and junior, played important roles . . . And one more friend must be mentioned," Blackmun said, "Sister Mary Brigh at Saint Marys. So cooperative, so helpful, so instructive."

In the face of enormous challenges, Methodists and colleagues reorganized the depleted Kahler facilities. Among the prime movers was a dynamic group of Rochester women who created a hospital auxiliary. True to form, it was Ralph Jester who sparked the idea of an RMH auxiliary. At his invitation, an auxiliary director from the American Hospital Association spoke to the RMH board. Several spouses of board members took the challenge, among them Dottie Blackmun and Billie Needham. Others soon joined them.

Mary Kahler Hench, wife of Nobel laureate Philip Hench, M.D., hosted the group's first meeting. "We wanted the event to be beautiful, optimistic," Billie Needham recalled. "A couple of us stripped our flower gardens of all their blooms and took them to the meeting . . . only to find that Mary's garden was full of blooms. Indoors and outdoors was a sea of flowers."

"We simply started by assuming we'd do everything," recalled Dottie Blackmun, the auxiliary's first president. "We didn't know much about an auxiliary or what went into running a hospital. What we did have was a tremendous ambition for it to succeed." Billie Needham remembered the stark hospital offices and bleak nurses' lounge. "Dottie Blackmun saw a great need to make offices look less like a business and more like a caring organization. We began by making drapes for all the offices and redecorated the nurses' lounge."

Writing letters or running errands for patients, staffing an information desk, reassuring anxious relatives, baking cookies for patients and staff, no job was too obscure, difficult, or distasteful for a volunteer to do. Kay Batchelder, who served twice as president of RMH auxiliary, commented on her predecessors. "These women were fearless risk takers, very smart and very persistent. It's not surprising that many of us are proud to follow that tradition."

Sister Mary Brigh viewed the RMH Auxiliary as a model for a similar organization at Saint Marys. With that in mind, she invited 35

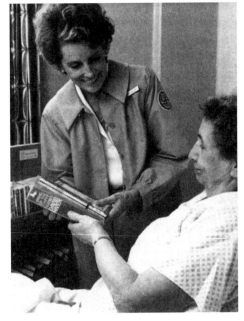

Auxilian/volunteer Sarah Waller visiting a patient with a bedside book cart. (From Caring, Summer 1988, p 4. Rochester, MN: Saint Marys Hospital.)

women to tea early in 1958. In Rochester's relatively small community, the meeting was a gathering of friends and neighbors. Dottie Blackmun and Priscilla Randall joined them to speak about the RMH Auxiliary. Concentrating on organization, programs, and fund-raising, they offered suggestions based on their experience. Sister Mary Brigh facilitated a spirited discussion. At the end of the meeting, 32 enthusiastic women volunteered as charter members of the new Saint Marys Hospital Auxiliary.

Mary Baldes, the auxiliary's president, hosted the first meeting where

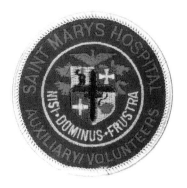

Insignia of the Saint Marys Hospital Auxiliary/Volunteers. (From Mayo Magazine, Summer 2005, p 57. Rochester, MN: Mayo Foundation for Medical Education and Research.)

members elected officers and formed committees. After defining their goals, auxilians established three initial service areas: assisting the patient library and pediatrics, serving as hostesses to newly admitted patients, and promoting fund-raising activities. Determined to make a difference, Saint Marys' auxilians embraced their new mission.

Two months later, the *Saint Marys News Bulletin* carried a front-page article praising the auxiliary. "Every once in a while something comes into our lives and so fills a need we can hardly conceive or even recall what our lives had been without it." The article went on to announce the auxiliary's newest service—the Coffee Cup. "We felt that relatives of patients, critically ill or in surgery, needed a cup of coffee and a bit of refreshment," explained Mary Baldes, "So we asked Sister Mary Brigh for a refreshment cart. The next day we were astonished when she offered us this room." The attractive Coffee Cup had no end of patrons—families, staff, and visitors. Auxilians contributed their earnings to hospital projects and patient needs. Over the years, the auxiliary created several variations of the Coffee Cup, among them, the coffee cart in the Francis and Mary Brigh Buildings and Hostess Service for intensive care areas.

Saint Marys Hospital auxilians soon took on other initiatives. In their first years of operation, patient visiting hours were restricted and hospitalizations lasted much longer. Conveniences taken for granted today, such as vending machines and the gift shop, were not available; nor did patients have telephones in their rooms. Auxilians created a Visiting Service and an Errand

Service. Volunteers visited patients and wrote letters for those far from home or unable to use their hands. Auxilians in the Errand Service helped patients with personal business and ran errands inside and outside the hospital. Volunteers offered a short order food service and, on occasion, prepared foods for patients in their homes.

Ginny Good, a charter member, recalled, "We often went to work with a little trepidation and not much bravado. There were times when, looking back, we seemed a little primitive organizationally. But they were great times, fun times. We were small, the hospital was not as large as it is now and our relationship with each other and with the Sisters was a lot like a family relationship. The important thing is that we served others. We also had fun—and we survived!"

Sister Lauren Weinandt, who came to Saint Marys from the novitiate in 1956, served as executive secretary to Sister Mary Brigh, and later Sister Generose Gervais. Her responsibilities included assisting the Auxiliary. Asked if she were the auxiliary coordinator, she quickly responded, "Sister Mary Brigh took the lead with the Auxiliary, as did Sister Generose in her administration. The door was always open to Auxilians." Sister Lauren's contribution, however, was significant, processing membership applications, figuring volunteer hours, and typing the monthly newsletter.

The "Pinkettes," the auxiliary's teen group, named Sister Lauren honorary member. Now called the "Young Volunteers," these women and men serve throughout the medical center. The organization's newsletter featured comments by teen volunteer Toni Brech, who served in Saint Marys Hospital. "Volunteering for me is a way to give back to the community for all that it has done for us. This allows me to meet new people who have the same interests as I do."

Saint Marys Auxiliary became involved with almost every aspect of hospital life. Auxilians in the Picture Cart Service offered patients a choice of pictures for their rooms. Volunteers brought musical entertainment and current events to the psychiatric floor. In 1973 the gift shop opened, providing a pleasant diversion and a welcome service. Gift shop earnings, distributed within Saint Marys, assist with patient needs, hospital projects, and the nursing scholarship fund.

In 1980, the organization created the position of "auxiliary coordinator." Sherri Wagner served as first coordinator, followed by Phyllis Hosking, and currently Susan Pronk. Working closely with the Auxiliary Board, they supported auxiliary members and guided activities.

Phyllis Hosking, coordinator from 1985 to 2001, reflected on her experiences. "Our volunteers, like many Rochester people, have a sensitivity for people who are hurting. Far from home, they often just need to talk with someone. Initially most of our members were married women who didn't work outside the home. Over time, as women went back to the workforce, we provided volunteer opportunities that fit their schedules. Increasingly, during my years as coordinator, hospital departments wanted to be more user-friendly. We helped develop several programs, such as the Emergency Room Service where volunteers interface with families and patients in the waiting room. This program and others like it reflect an emphasis on hospitality that recalls the auxiliary's first programs."

Among her accomplishments, Phyllis Hosking hired Ann Freund, the auxiliary's first secretary. Ann, who relates to volunteers and the medical center as a whole, commented on the appreciation she hears for volunteer services. She spoke of the Surgical Messenger Service. "The service keeps families informed about patients in surgery. It's very challenging, but volunteers don't seem to miss a beat. They make an enormous difference to families and staff." Asked about her own position, Ann responded, "Everyone wants to be here. That's one of the reasons I like coming to work."

The current coordinator, Susan Pronk, commented on auxiliary membership. "From my experience every volunteer seems to have the same heart set—they all want to be of service. Our members, who include men and women, consistently number 300 or more. Volunteers join for a variety of reasons, for example, Saint Marys retired employees have a strong allegiance to Saint Marys Hospital. They want to keep connected. Others join out of appreciation for the care that relatives received at Saint Marys. Marie Aaberg, whose family members were Saint Marys patients, took a sabbatical from teaching to join the auxiliary. Marie was from Mankato, Minnesota, about fifty miles away; she drove a considerable distance, as do several others members. Marie is now Mayo's coordinator of Young Volunteers."

Susan spoke of her appreciation for the Franciscan volunteers. "They not only serve in specific areas, but also fill in when we need help in a hurry. Sisters who retire from the auxiliary stay involved by making items, such as baby booties and blankets, for the gift shop." Susan made special mention of Sister Vera Klinkhammer, who "broke the record this year with 20,000 lifetime hours."

At 95, Sister Vera, in her high heels, visits patients every day of the week. "Patients love to see her coming," noted Susan, "so does the staff—she keeps them on their toes." For many years, Sister Vera, a retired nursing supervisor, visited patients with her blood sister, Sister Gildas Klinkhammer, until Sister Gildas died at one hundred and one. Recently she recalled Sister Gildas' response to staff members who said they didn't have to work on weekends. "Patients," she informed them, "are sick on weekends too!" In the evenings Sister Vera walks the hospital corridors collecting unused items that she recycles and gives to local, national, and international charities. "Sister Vera is truly a legend."

Bonnie Jean Maher, a volunteer since 1989, expressed a theme that echoes across the auxiliary, "I receive much more from my interactions with patients and families than I could ever give." Bonnie, like her peers, makes a significant contribution. Twice president of the auxiliary, she served 6 years on the executive committee in addition to her weekly hospital service. Asked if this was a burden, Bonnie quickly replied, "Not at all—everyone wants to be here—we all work together for the same purpose, service to others. The Franciscan spirit that began with the Sisters continues to bring many rewards for all of us."

ENDNOTES

Page 131   *Rochester Post-Bulletin* October 1, 1956, p 1.

Pages 131-132   **Martin Maurice J:** *A View of the First 50 Years of Psychiatry and Psychology at the Mayo Clinic.* **Rochester, MN: Mayo Foundation for Medical Education and Research, 1997, pp 9, 11, 19.**

Page 132   *The Courier* October 4, 1956, p 1.

Pages 132-133   Interviews with J. M. Stickney, M.D. and Sister M. Immaculata. **In: Dusbabek MH:** *The Contributions of Sister M. Domitilla DuRocher, O.S.F. to Nursing, 1920-1939.* **Unpublished dissertation. Catholic University of America, Washington, DC, 1962, p 37.**
Mayo's response to Sister Domitilla's request for a psychiatry unit in 1935.

Page 133   **Mayo Clinic Section of Neurology, Annual Reports, 1944, 1945.**

                 Psychiatry at Saint Marys. *Caring* **Spring 1978, p 3.**
Quote from Dr. Howard P. Rome.

                 Change About Thinking in Nurses Training Described by Sister Julié. *Rochester Post-Bulletin* **April 22, 1950.**

Page 134   **Martin (p 29).**

                 Interview with Marjorie Habenicht Overby, February 16, 2003.

                 Interview with Sister Mary Lynch, February 15, 2006.

Page 135   **Yesterday: the First "Emergency Rooms."** *Caring* **Winter 1981, p 8.**

                 Interview with Patricia Hooley, March 7, 2005.

Page 136   Interview with Charlotte Carey, February 17, 2005.

Page 137   **Yesterday: the "First Emergency Rooms" (p 8).**
Quotes from Marlene Staley.

                 Interview with Sister Regina Buskowiak, February 15, 2006.

Page 138   **Harold A. Wente, M.D.: Unpublished memoirs.**

Interview with C. Dale Rustad, June 7, 2006.

Page 139   **C. Dale Rustad:** *Mayo Magazine* **Autumn 2004, p 8.**

Pages 139-140   Interviews with Sandy Zimmerman Hanson, June 1, 2006 and July 14, 2006.

Presentation to Mayo Finance Department, December 9, 2004.

Page 141   **Opitz JL: The Early History of the Department of Physical Medicine and Rehabilitation, Mayo Clinic (1911-1935): The Root Departments. In:** *History of the Mayo Clinic Department of Physical Medicine and Rehabilitation, 1911-2002.* **Edited by JL Opitz, RW DePompolo. Rochester, MN: Mayo Foundation for Medical Education and Research, 2005, p 1.**

Interview with Robert W. DePompolo, M.D., February 16, 2005.

Pages 141-142   **Opitz JL: The Section on Physical Medicine (1942-1947): Chair, Frank H. Krusen, M.D. In:** *History of the Mayo Clinic Department of Physical Medicine and Rehabilitation, 1911-2002.* **Edited by JL Opitz, RW DePompolo, p 82.**

Page 142   **Opitz (pp 47, 56).**

Pages 142-143   Interview with Sister Regina Buskowiak, February 15, 2006.

Page 143   Interview with Sister Germaine Hullerman, August 10, 2005.

Interview with Claire E. Bender, M.D., August 14, 2003.

Holmes W: *Dedicated to Excellence: The Rochester Methodist Hospital Story.* **Rochester, MN: Rochester Methodist Hospital Foundation, 1984, p 43.**

Page 144   **Holmes (p 45).**

Pages 144-145   **Holmes (pp 66-71).**

Pages 145-146   **Holmes (pp 107-109).**

Pages 146-147   Interview with Kay Batchelder, August 1, 2006 and Kay Batchelder and Karen Ostrander, June 20, 2006.

Pages 147-148   *Saint Marys Hospital News Bulletin* **May 1958.**

Page 148   **The Saint Marys Hospital Auxiliary: Looking Back on 25 Years.** *Caring* **Spring 1983, p 4.**

Interviews with Sister Lauren Weinandt, May 15, 2006 and July 24, 2006.

Mayo Clinic Young Volunteers. **Rochester, MN: Mayo Foundation for Medical Education and Research, March/April 2005, p 3.**

Page 149   Interviews with Phyllis Hosking, June 16, 2006 and July 16, 2006.

Interview with Ann Freund, August 7, 2006.

Interview with Susan Pronk, August 7, 2006.

Pages 149-150   Interview with Sister Vera Klinkhammer, August 10, 2005.

Page 150   Interview with Bonnie Maher, August 4, 2006.

CHAPTER 8

Eminent Surgeons

The distinguished surgeon, O. T. "Jim" Clagett, M.D., wrote a history of general surgery at Mayo. Personally self-effacing, Dr. Clagett did not understate Mayo's achievements. "It seems unlikely that any other group of surgeons at any institution anytime, anywhere contributed to surgery or influenced surgery as have the 43 surgeons who were on the surgical staff of the Mayo Clinic from 1900 to 1970."

This chapter focuses on the period 1940 to 1980, the time frame of the book. In the history of Mayo Clinic, the first surgeons—namely William Worrall Mayo, M.D., and his sons, William J. Mayo, M.D., and Charles H. Mayo, M.D. (Will and Charlie), were general surgeons. The chapter begins with general surgery and goes on to note the movement toward specialization for Mayo clinicians and surgeons. Mayo surgeons at Saint Marys Hospital developed specialized surgical procedures in several areas. Cardiac surgery and neurosurgery, with their unique historic connections to the hospital, are featured in this chapter.

The story of surgery, as Dr. Will Mayo noted, owed a great deal to timing. "Stress the unusual opportunity," he urged his biographer, "that existed in the time, the place, the general setup, not to be duplicated now." Infection was the surgeon's greatest nemesis. Even after a successful surgical procedure, septic infections invaded the patient's wounds and caused high fever and, many times, death. In 1867, Scottish surgeon Joseph Lister demonstrated that microorganisms caused surgical infections and that antisepsis could kill them. Dr. Will and Dr. Charlie used wet antisepsis, which evolved into the aseptic technique. As a result, patient death rates at Saint Marys Hospital averaged only 2.1% within the first 4 years, an almost unheard of rate.

Fired with ambition to create a surgical center on a level with hospitals in the eastern United States, the Mayos kept abreast of new developments. "We were a green crew and we knew it," Dr. Will admitted. One at a time, over several years, the Mayo brothers made extended visits to medical centers in this country and abroad. They brought back new ideas and shared them with the Sisters, who were equally committed to developing in their areas of practice. The Mayos and Franciscans set standards for excellence and teamwork that continue to inspire the institution today.

"Working in their remote location, far from urban centers and nearby competitors," writes surgeon W. F. Braasch, M.D., "the Mayos performed some operations by the hundreds, or even by the thousands." In 1905, the *Olmsted County Democrat* observed, "Practically no European surgeon of note crosses the country without coming to Rochester." During operations, the brothers always discussed their procedures for the benefit of visitors, who came from different areas of the country and from around the world. "As the numbers of visiting surgeons increased, movable, elevated metal stands were positioned to allow a better view of an operation from the sidelines. Over the operating tables, large adjustable mirrors provided a complete view of the operating field." In response to increasing demand for advanced training, the Clinic established Mayo's graduate school of medicine in 1915, "the country's first graduate program in clinical medicine."

The Doctors Mayo encouraged their staff to develop clinical specialties. In 1924, Dr. Will Mayo wrote: "Specialization has come to stay. The enormous amount of learning now available in surgery makes successful generalization so difficult of accomplishment that to become a competent all-round surgeon is almost impossible." Individually, physicians pursued particular areas of medicine and worked together to provide superior patient care.

In 1897, 8 years after Saint Marys opened, the Mayos performed 915 operations. The number grew to 1,823 by 1900, to 3,154 by 1903, and 4,770 by 1906—more than any hospital in the United States. Unprecedented growth created problems of overcrowding and prompted a series of Mayo requests for hospital additions. By 1912, five new additions increased the hospital's capacity to 300 beds and six operating rooms with galleries for observation. In 1922, at a cost of 2.25 million dollars, Sister Joseph supervised the construction of the surgical pavilion, later named in her honor. Acclaimed "the most up to date surgical pavilion in the entire world," the Joseph Building doubled the number of hospital beds to 600.

Until 1922, 33 years after its founding, Saint Marys was a primarily surgical hospital. The demand for surgical beds left no room for patients with exclusively medical problems. The Joseph Building, devoted entirely to surgery and surgery beds, created an opportunity to serve medical patients in other areas of the hospital.

Ten years later, Doris Unland, just out of high school, boarded a train in the Colorado Rockies that brought her to Rochester and Saint Marys School of Nursing. She traveled this distance, in her words, "because Saint Marys was simply the best." During her 45 years in the operating room, Doris became a legendary surgical nurse and supervisor. "I worked," Doris declared, "with the finest surgeons in the world." She credited much of her own expertise to the Sisters who served as head nurses in every operating room when she came to Saint Marys.

The duties of surgical nurses in those days went beyond assisting with operations. They sewed caps and masks, folded and sterilized linens, washed, patched, and sterilized rubber gloves. After washing, boiling, and rinsing gauze packs dipped in saline solution, they hung them out to dry on the Joseph building balconies. By the mid 1950s, linen suppliers and packaged surgical gloves eliminated most of this work. By that time, however, other aspects of surgery had become more difficult.

"The period of World War II was probably the busiest time surgically we've ever had," Doris Unland recalled. "So many physicians were called into the service that those of us who were left worked harder than ever. It was not unusual for one surgeon to do 13 to 15 procedures a day, sometimes as many as 20, and to work six days a week."

Sister Paula Leopold, who called Doris Unland "mentor and friend," served as a young nurse in surgery during World War II. Like Doris, she worked under Sister William "Bill" Fischenich. Reputedly, Sister William never stopped to rest and expected the same of others. Mayo surgeon, James T. Priestly, M.D., paid tribute to the Sisters with a dash of hyperbole, "In those days, a nun was always head nurse. These nuns always worked 24 to 26 hours per day with no complaints." Sister Paula quickly caught the spirit. Surgeries began at 7:00 in the morning and she remembered days when they finished at 11:00 in the evening. "The next day we began again at 7:00 and remained until all surgeries were completed, perhaps twelve or fourteen hours at a stretch. We were young, help was very short, and we did what we were asked to do."

One evening, after Stewart W. Harrington, M.D., operated on a small child, he told Sister William the child must have a special duty night nurse.

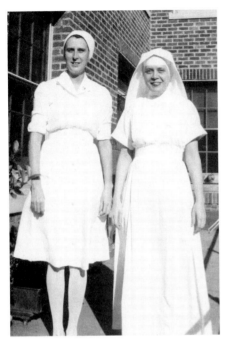

Doris Unland and Sister Paula Leopold, surgery supervisors. (From Saint Marys Hospital Archives.)

No special duty nurse was available so Sister Paula got the assignment. "I was terrified but of course I did it. I was afraid I'd fall asleep and something would happen to the child. To keep awake, I stood by the side of the bed all night long and watched the child breathe. I don't think I was ever happier to see the sun rise and hear the day nurses report for duty."

The dedication of Sister Paula and others like her impressed Donald C. McIlrath, M.D., who came to Rochester as a surgical fellow in 1957. "Before I came to Mayo, I worked in or visited many hospitals. I was amazed by the operation of Saint Marys Hospital. Every operation hummed with talented staffs, who obviously were dedicated to the welfare of every patient. The secret of this success was due, without question, to the Sisters of Saint Francis who held supervisory positions in administration, medical and surgical stations, operating suites, laundry, food service, and housekeeping. The Sisters performed their respective roles with confidence, dignity, and incredible effort, which set the pace and tone for all hospital employees, fellows, and staff of Mayo Clinic."

Dr. McIlrath's 5-year surgical fellowship program was a rigorous, intense experience based on the preceptor model in combination with research in the basic sciences. Typically, surgical fellows began their day at 5:00 a.m. In addition to dressing wounds of postsurgical patients, they brought surgical patients on carts to the operating rooms by 7:15 a.m.—no exceptions— and the day was only beginning. As a fellow in the 1950s, Dr. McIlrath received a monthly stipend of $75 to $100.

Because so many surgeons wished to spend their entire careers at Mayo, new staff appointments were relatively rare. Nevertheless, Dr. McIlrath was appointed to the surgical staff in 1962. "His major field of interest is surgery of the gastrointestinal tract," wrote Dr. Clagett. "He is an unusually

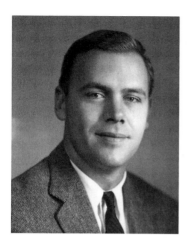

Donald C. McIlrath, M.D., began his Mayo career as a surgical resident in 1957 and joined the staff in 1962. (From Dr. McIlrath's collection.)

skilled technical surgeon who performs difficult operations with precision and ease."

Now a member of the Mayo Clinic's private group practice, Dr. McIlrath received an annual salary, as did all his physician peers and indeed all Mayo employees. Dr. Clagett, a surgeon, and William "Bill" McConahey, M.D., an internist, assessed the advantages Mayo's private group practice for the individual physician, the institution, and above all, the patient.

"No surgeon at the Clinic," wrote Dr. Clagett, "regardless of his fame or the number of surgeries he performed, became wealthy from his Clinic salary. However, monetary returns were never an important concern to Mayo Clinic surgeons. They enjoyed a unique environment to live and work in. They were provided with the best possible facilities and equipment . . . Highly competent consultants and specialists were readily available . . . to help solve some unexpected problems. The whole atmosphere of the institution stimulated one's best possible efforts in all aspects of surgical practice, research, and teaching . . . And most importantly, every surgeon had the great satisfaction of knowing that the money he earned for the institution beyond his own salary would be used exclusively to provide funds for research and for the education of future surgeons."

Dr. McConahey spoke of "standing on the shoulders of giants," whose altruism and caring for the patient first were powerful examples. "The fact that we were all on salary made it easy to ask surgeons for their opinion on the advisability of surgery. I had no question that their motivation would be for the good of the patient and not to make more money. I knew that surgeons got more money than I did, but I received a good salary and the benefits that I received as a staff member meant a good deal."

Dr. McIlrath served at Saint Marys as a staff general surgeon from 1962 to 1977. He recalled the scrub nurses "who were so knowledgeable that it was rarely necessary to ask for an instrument because they were ready to pass an instrument before you even thought you needed it. They often stood for 11 or 12 hours and performed with the same efficiency. He remembered nights when Doris Unland, who could see the OR lights from her home near the hospital, came back to work to see if she could help. Dr. McIlrath also spoke of nursing supervisors on the floors. "I especially remember Jane Campion (Sister Richaea), who was in charge of a nursing floor. It seemed she was always there, knew the details of every patient's care, and was in touch with the patients' family members."

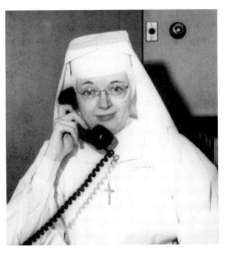

As nursing supervisor, Jane Campion (Sister Richaea) "knew the details of every patient's care." (From Saint Marys Hospital Archives.)

Surgical opportunities and challenges increased dramatically during World War II for Dr. Jim Clagett. Unlike most of his colleagues, Dr. Clagett was not called to military service. He and the few surgeons who remained at Mayo heroically served record numbers of patients. During these years Dr. Clagett incorporated wartime advances in thoracic and cardiovascular surgery. Speaking of himself, he wrote, "Because Dr. Clagett was at the right place at the right time, he was able to participate actively and contribute to practically every aspect of the rapid growth and development of thoracic and cardiovascular surgery." At the 2005 celebration of Mayo's fifty years of cardiovascular surgery, thoracic surgeon Peter C. Pairolero, M.D., paid tribute to Dr. Clagett in a description of his colleague's pioneer work. Dr. Pairolero concluded, "I'm sure you'll agree, Jim Clagett was Mayo's first cardiovascular surgeon."

In response to the postwar demand for cardiovascular surgeries, Mayo appointed gifted Rochester native, John W. Kirklin, M.D., to the staff in 1950. Kirklin, who began a Mayo surgical fellowship in 1944, recalled his early interest in this specialty. "My fellow residents and I filled pages of notebooks with drawings and plans of how we would close ventricular septal defects and repair the Tetralogy of Fallot once science gave us a method to get inside the heart."

Scientists worldwide worked to design a device that allowed surgeons to operate "under direct vision in a bloodless field within the opened heart." Surgeon John H. Gibbon, M.D., of Philadelphia's Jefferson Medical College began such a project in 1937 with partial funding from Thomas J. Watson of IBM. In 1953, after 16 years, Dr. Gibbon used the Gibbon-IBM pump oxygenator to successfully complete one open-heart procedure. Two subsequent patients died, however, and Gibbon made no further attempts. In the meantime, Mayo scientists continued in their efforts.

In 1952, Dr. Kirklin assembled a team of experts to develop a cardiac surgical program for the clinical application of the mechanical pump-oxygenator. Mayo physicians, surgeons, and scientists from distinct but complementary disciplines collaborated on this singular effort. After Kirklin obtained blueprints of the Gibbon-IBM pump-oxygenator, Mayo engineers refined and modified the basic design. In two and a half years, they successfully developed a pump-oxygenator. "By 1955," wrote Kirklin, "we were in a position to proceed with clinical application." The clinical and engineering achievements of Dr. Kirklin and his team were astonishing. Within 3 years they developed a cardiac clinical program and the pump-oxygenator. Anesthesiologist Emerson A. Moffitt, M.D., who assisted in this effort, called Mayo's multidisciplinary achievement, "another Manhattan Project."

Dr. Kirklin and his team introduced open-heart surgery at Mayo in 1955. The first operation, performed at Methodist Hospital, closed a ventricular septal defect in a 5-year-old girl. Soon after the event, *Medical Horizons*, a nationally televised series with an audience of 6 to 9 million, featured Mayo's new open-heart surgery program as the first segment of its 26-week series.

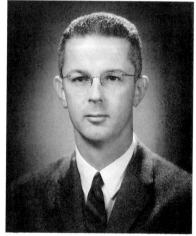

In addition to the "steady stream of scientific presentations," Mayo historian John L. Graner, M.D., credits the rapid increase of cardiac referrals to *Medical Horizons* and other media coverage. This increase prompted Dr. Kirklin to look to Saint Marys Hospital with its larger facilities as a new base for the program. Surgery supervisor Sister Merici Maher, who had worked with Dr. Kirklin, remembered his casual question, "Sister, would you happen to know anyone who could help us bring the open-heart surgery program to Saint Marys?" Sister Merici told him she thought she knew someone. Subsequently, she spoke with hospital

John W. Kirklin, M.D., and his team of experts introduced open-heart surgery at Mayo in 1955. (From Mayo Clinic Archives.)

administrator Sister Mary Brigh, who responded, "I don't see any problem with that."

Hospital annals of August 15, 1956 note, "Agreement reached by all. Cardiovascular surgery will move to Saint Marys." Sister Merici, then cardiac surgical supervisor, noted, "I was privileged to work with Dr. Kirklin and his team in the early years of cardiac development. Every day was a new experience." Sister Merici later described her experience as supervisor of the operating room. "The surgeons I worked with were men of integrity, compassion, and real gentlemen. Of course, there were conflicts, but we resolved them in a constructive way. Surgeons, anesthesiologists, nurse anesthetists, operating room nurses, and technicians worked well together."

Sister Carmen Sonnek (Sister Pierce), trained by Sister Merici, followed her as cardiac scrub nurse and supervisor. "With the first cardiac surgeries," Sister Carmen remembered, "we would be in the operating room 10 or 12 hours at a time. No day was the same. It was an intense experience and I quickly learned the technical skills necessary to anticipate the surgeon's needs. It was also a difficult time. We lost a number of our patients in those years. Open-heart surgery initially concentrated on congenital heart defects and most of our patients were infants and children whose parents brought them to Mayo as a last resort.

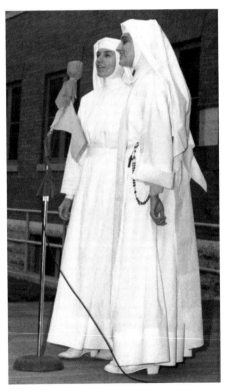

"Sister Merici and I shared on-call duty for emergencies every other day, 24 hours a day. I believe I was on call 12 years of my 14 years in surgery. During the on-call time, we had to stay close to the phone. I spent free time working on art projects on the back porch of Saint Mary's convent and listened to every kind of music, from opera and symphonies

Surgery supervisors and talented singers Sister Carmen Sonnek (Sister Pierce, left) and Sharon Ann Stanton (Sister Pilar, right) entertain employees at a Saint Marys Hospital Fall BBQ. (From Saint Marys Hospital Archives.)

to jazz and country. Working on projects, listening to music, and singing in the Sisters' choir helped get me through those intense years."

Under Dr. Kirklin's leadership, the expanding department of cardio-vascular surgery added new staff: F. Henry Ellis, Jr., M.D., Dwight C. McGoon, M.D., Robert B. Wallace, M.D., and Gordon K. Danielson, M.D. Nursing staff also increased, among them Sister Cynthia Howe, who served as scrub nurse for Dr. Wallace for 15 years. Committed to assisting new employees, Sister Cynthia created resources to help them develop their skills. "I wrote a manual for new employees who came to surgery without training. To help inexperienced technicians I color-coded the items surgeons requested during surgery. This allowed them to look for colors rather than trying to read instructions when they were under great tension." "And," she added with a grin, "it worked!"

In mid-August 1956, Sister Mary Brigh wrote the directive for the creation of an intensive care unit (ICU), among the first in the country. "A special nursing unit will be set up in the 12-bed north wing of 3-Domitilla for the early post-operative care of these patients, both for children and adults. Sister Elizabeth Gillis (Sister Maristella) will be in charge. Staff will be nine professional graduates, four vocational graduates, and four nurse aides. Patients will come to the Unit directly from sur-gery and stay as long as the doctor directs. No private duty nurses will be assigned to the unit."

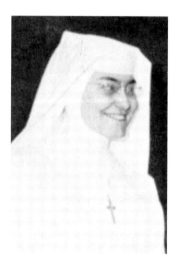

Later, Sister Mary Brigh told an audience, "Emergency treatment may mean the differ-ence between life and death" for patients who survived open-heart surgery. "The intensive care unit," she explained, "concentrates in one area the patients needing expert care, the personnel qualified to give that care, and the special equipment needed to give it, in a manner that no ordinary hospital has or can duplicate."

Sister Elizabeth, 24 years old at the time, vividly recalled her ICU experience almost 50 years later. "In September 1956 Sister Mary Brigh asked me to assume leadership of a ten-or twelve-bed unit, which would open on 3 Domitilla. Within the month, four of us, Sister

Sister Elizabeth Gillis served as head nurse in Saint Marys Hospital's first intensive care unit. (From Saint Marys Hospital News Bulletin, Vol. XXI, no. 2, February 1962.)

Mary Brigh, nursing director Sister Florence Zweber (Sister Aquinette), Dr. Kirklin, and I met several times.

"We wrote the directions/protocol for the care of post-operative patients according to three standards of care: Constant Care; Intermediate Care; and Regular Care in 3 Domitilla proper where Sister Maeve Cashman (Marge Cashman Gallagher) was nursing supervisor. Maeve and I had a wonderful working relationship. Our nurses were outstanding, but none of us knew anything about caring for cardiac surgery patients. I went up to the University of Minnesota for one day and observed surgery, another day I went to Methodist Hospital where Dr. Kirklin first performed open-heart surgery. And that was it.

"Constant Care pertained to patients coming to the unit immediately after surgery. They were checked every fifteen minutes for blood pressure, pulse, respiration, intravenous fluids (chest discharge). This was all done manually; for example, the chest drainage equipment was on the floor and had to be read at eye level. I remember getting down on my hands and knees every 15 minutes to read at eye level. Intermediate patients were checked every hour, then every 2 hours, and subsequently went to the nursing floor in close proximity. There were no monitors. Oxygen was administered by mask or, in the case of children, by tent. We had no air conditioning. When patients spiked a temp, we used sponges to bathe them with alcohol and ice to bring it down.

"One nurse per patient, each room had 2 patients and therefore two nurses on constant duty. A resident physician always accompanied each patient from surgery. The rooms were very crowded with equipment on the floors rather than in the walls as it is now. Charts stood at the end of the bed on stands, so that we could observe the patient carefully and note each observation by hand every 15 minutes. There were no machines to tell us how a patient was doing, it was all observation and we had to be acutely observant. We were learning all the time, and so were the doctors.

"Many days five patients came from surgery to that small unit—we scrambled to care for them. I don't know how the surgeons did it, hours and hours of surgery. Surgeons at this time were Drs. Kirklin and F.H. Ellis. Dr. McGoon joined them a little later. I had heard about this doctor who was coming from Johns Hopkins. The first time I saw him I noticed an unfamiliar figure standing in the corner of the room. He was observing what was going on with a patient who had just come down from surgery. When I went over to him, he said, 'Sister, I'm Dwight McGoon.'

"Dr. McGoon was an outstanding person and physician. One of the kindest, gentlest physicians I've ever met. In his first weeks at Mayo he didn't do surgery, but was responsible for coordinating the cardiac ICU. The nurses got to know him well and we had great respect for him—he was compassionate, skilled with patients, extremely helpful to nursing staff. I remember one of the nurses commenting, 'He must have some faults. I bet he leaves the cap off the toothpaste!' Dr. McGoon stayed in the unit for 12 hours at a time, not even leaving for meals. I went to the convent dining room for food and brought him a tray. He ate in the doctors' conference room.

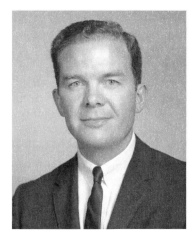

Cardiac surgeon Dwight C. McGoon, M.D., was an inspiration to staff and patients alike. (From Mayo Clinic Archives.)

"We had many sick patients and deaths were not uncommon. After a surgery, I'd first see that patients were settled in their rooms, then go to the waiting room, and speak with the family. In the case of death, I met with families in a small, private room. A surgeon would join us. I remember one Sunday when there were three deaths. I had already met with two families and was on my way to visit with the third, when I met Sister Generose in the hall. 'I don't know if I can do this,' I told her. Sister Generose took my hand and said, 'You'll be okay.'"

Caring for patients who came to the nursing floor from ICU was an intense learning experience for staff. "In the first three or four months of open-heart surgery," Sister Maeve recalled, "Dr. Kirklin was committed to educating the nursing staff. Before the day shift began, about 6:45, he came to the floor to teach us, with detailed specifics, about the heart and the principles of good cardiac care. His purpose was to inform us and to create a good working team. It was an invaluable experience as we began to work with these patients."

Teamwork was a key component of Mayo's cardiac program. "The teamwork involved in such surgery is astonishing," notes Mayo historian Victor Johnson, M.D. "There are clinicians, cardiologists, radiologists, clinical pathologists, anesthesiologists, residents, nurses, dietitians, by-pass machine operators, social workers and perhaps more." Years later, Dr. Dwight McGoon commented that each person "holds a key post. The cardiac surgeon plays a major part, but even with the training, hard work, and discipline that he must master, he is but a leader and not a soloist."

Young and relatively inexperienced, clinical dietitian Rosemary White was asked to serve cardiac patients. "It was a dramatic experience for me to serve in cardiac care," she recalled, "Patients were on restricted sodium diets and it was critical that they maintained this restriction after they left the hospital. The nurses and doctors, who were wonderful to work with, strongly supported the importance of the diet. When I'd visit patients, who would much rather see their doctor than hear from me, the physician would tell the patient, 'We can talk later. You listen to the diet instructions and I'll come back.' I particularly appreciated Dr. McGoon—his ability to relate to all of us and help us work as a team was outstanding. I also had unstinting support from the dietary supervisor, Sister Victorine [Honerman], who went to great lengths to assist patients and staff."

"The close and continuing collaboration of physicians, surgeons, scientists, and others from distinct but complementary disciplines," writes Dr. Graner, distinguished Mayo's heart program. "Moreover, each individual rapidly gained extensive experience due to the large number of cardiac patients referred to the Clinic." The concept of the Coronary Care Unit (CCU), noted in the next chapter, evolved largely from this multidisciplinary experience.

In the story of Mayo's eminent surgeons, neurologic surgery, unlike open-heart surgery, had a long history at Saint Marys Hospital. In an article marking 100 years of neurologic surgery, neurologists Robert J. Spinner, M.D., Nayef R.F. Al-Rodhan, M.D., and David G. Piepgras, M.D., trace its history and development. "Beginning with a single surgeon performing a modest number of cases each year, the practice of neurologic surgery at the Mayo Clinic has grown to become one of the largest neurosurgical services in North America." Dr. Spinner's article, along with memoirs and interviews with nursing supervisors, Sister Amadeus Klein and Catherine "Kate" Towey, provide a framework for this section on neurosurgery.

Early records attest to neurologic procedures performed by Dr. Charlie Mayo at Saint Marys Hospital as early as 1891. In 1907, when Emil H. Beckman, M.D., became Dr. Charlie's assistant, prevailing opinion considered neurosurgical cases hopeless. Dr. Beckman, however, developed a major interest in neurosurgery. After Dr. Beckman's untimely death in 1917, Alfred W. Adson, M.D., then a surgical fellow, was asked to join the Clinic.

As a general surgeon, Dr. Adson "took whatever neurological cases came his way." Asked to focus on neurological surgery, he was initially

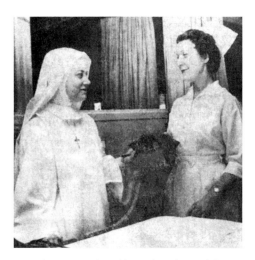

Nursing supervisor Sister Amadeus Klein (left) confers with head nurse Nina Bowers. (From Rochester Post-Bulletin, January 31, 1958. Used with permission.)

reluctant. After five neurosurgical procedures, however, he changed his mind. The last procedure, Dr. Adson's first laminectomy, was memorable. "As luck would have it," notes Spinner, "the procedure was observed by visiting physicians from the British army (Sir Barkley Monyhan), the French army (Dr. Duvall), and the Italian army (Dr. Bastinelli)."In an effort to relieve the strain on the young surgeon, Drs. Will and Charlie Mayo urged the distinguished guests to join them for lunch. "The army surgeons insisted on staying," recalled Dr. Adson, "so what did the Doctors Will and Charlie do but join the group." Fortunately, the procedure and recovery were uneventful. "It was this case that prompted Sir Barkley to say that he had seen a high school boy doing neurosurgery at the Mayo Clinic, referring to Dr. Adson's youthful appearance (he was 30 years old at the time)."

Five years later, in 1921, Dr. Will Mayo asked Dr. Adson to "develop the specialty of neurosurgery at the Mayo Clinic." He agreed with three conditions: "1) that neurosurgery should encompass facets of surgery relative to the nervous system; 2) that neurosurgery should be independent from the Division of Surgery; and 3) that neurological surgeons should have the same financial benefits as the general surgeons as the Mayo Clinic. Dr. Mayo agreed."

"Dr. Adson was strict and demanded quality care from both the medical and nursing staff." Sister Amadeus commented, "He showed warmth for his patients and concern for the circumstances they faced. I remember the time he visited a young man who was paralyzed after severing his spine in a hunting accident. Dr. Adson called me over. 'Sister, this man planned to be married this weekend. He is very ill but they still want to be married. Call the preacher and arrange for their marriage in his hospital room.'"

As chairman of neurosurgery from 1917 to 1946, Dr. Adson added new staff to meet growing numbers of patients with neurological conditions. Among those he hired, three men followed him as chairmen of the department, Winchell McK. Craig, M.D., J. Grafton Love, M.D., and Collin S. MacCarty, M.D.

Dr. Craig, who headed the department from 1946 to 1955, developed a reputation "for tackling neurosurgical cases that were difficult because of either technical or physiological problems." Sister Amadeus later noted such an instance. "We visited a seriously ill patient on rounds who seemed to be making little or no progress. Dr. Craig carefully reviewed the record and told me, 'Sister, stop all IVs, oxygen, and medication, but give her good nursing care.' Minutes later the first assistant approached me. 'Sister, we can't do this!' I explained that Dr. Craig used this approach to find a base line and determine what the body could do for its own recovery. The assistant was relieved, but somewhat skeptical. The next day the patient showed a little improvement and we resumed treatment; later the patient recovered enough to go home."

Like Sister Amadeus, other Sisters were closely associated with neurosurgery, among them, Sister Theodora Mikolai. Sister Theodora, who came to the congregation in 1897, was among the last Sisters to learn nursing from Edith Graham Mayo. She became a surgical nurse and continued in that position for more than 50 years. "We put in some long days," she recalled. "After surgery we always cleaned the operating rooms. Then, in the afternoon we boiled surgical gloves, cut surgical sponges, and even made sutures from horsehair. I remember how Sister Joseph used to take hair from the horses we had. We'd get enough to make a roll and then we'd soak it in strong soap for a week before boiling it to be used in surgery."

Later, Sister Theodora was in charge of spinal taps and taught this procedure to many of the physicians. Exacting about technique and frugal with materials, Sister Theodora was a strong personality. Some physicians found her difficult; others like neurosurgeon Henry W. Dodge Jr., M.D., admired and respected her. When Dr.

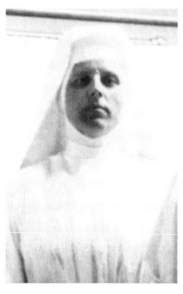

A surgical nurse for over 50 years, Sister Theodora Mikolai was a mentor for young surgeons who learned spinal tap procedures under her direction. (From Saint Marys Hospital Archives.)

Dodge left Rochester, he gave Sister Theodora his country estate "for the use of the Sisters." Gaelic Grove, as it is called, remains a favorite gathering place for Franciscans—thanks to Dr. Dodge and Sister Theodora.

An avid reader, Sister Theodora found copies of her favorite newspapers, the *Wall Street Journal* and the *New York Times*, and read them on Sunday afternoons. In later years, she spent many hours in chapel praying for patients, staff, and the needs of the world gleaned from her beloved newspapers. In 1986, after 89 years at Saint Marys Hospital, Sister Theodora died quietly at the age of 106.

Dr. Collin MacCarty, who also had high regard and personal affection for Sister Theodora, chaired the department from 1963 to 1975. Dr. MacCarty was second in three generations of three MacCarty physicians to serve at Mayo. His father, William C. MacCarty, M.D., chaired the section on Surgical Pathology and his son, Robert L. MacCarty, M.D., is a Mayo radiologist. Dr. MacCarty grew up next to Saint Marys Hospital and later raised his own family in the same neighborhood. The MacCarty children knew the Sisters when they worked with chickens behind the hospital, tended the large vegetable gardens, and tapped hospital maple trees for syrup. Needless to say, the bond was strong between the MacCartys and the Franciscans.

Dr. MacCarty and the Sisters worked closely in the planning and construction of state-of-the-art neurologic facilities. With Sister Amadeus and the nursing staff he helped develop the hospital's first neurological ICU that opened in 1958. Subsequently, over a 3-year period, Dr. MacCarty led a group of Mayo physicians and engineers who researched and planned "the most modern neurosurgical operating rooms in the world." Sisters Mary Brigh and Generose worked with Saint Marys' legendary engineer, William "Bill" Cribbs, and his colleagues on the project. In 1963, the complex installation was completed. Recalling these accomplishments, Dr. MacCarty declared, "The Sisters knew just what we needed and spared no effort to get it done."

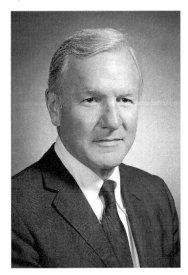

Collin S. MacCarty, M.D., the second in three generations of MacCarty physicians at Mayo, was a noted neurosurgeon. (From Mayo Clinic Archives.)

Dr. MacCarty was a pioneer in the 1960s in profound hypothermia for procedures on intracranial vascular disorders. At that time, neurosurgeons temporarily reduced blood flow to the brain while they operated on damaged nerves and brain tissue by dropping the body temperature as low as eighty-four degrees. The procedure required 8 to 14 hours of anesthesia time and demanded exclusive dedication by both the neurosurgeon and anesthesiologist. "The challenge provided by this revolutionary technique," writes anesthesiologist John D. Michenfelder, M.D., "spawned the introduction of clinical research into neurosurgical anesthesia at the Mayo Clinic."

Neurosurgical anesthesia had its roots 10 years earlier, when anesthesiologist John E. Osborn, M.D., focused on anesthesia for neurosurgery "in part because of his friendship with neurosurgeon Dr. Collin MacCarty." Though Dr. Osborn died prematurely of a brain tumor in 1957, other anesthesiologists, including Dr. Michenfelder, continued his mission. Their collaborative efforts established neuroanesthesia as a subspecialty at Mayo Clinic, the first of its kind in the United States.

Catherine "Kate" Towey was among the first nurses on the neuro ICU unit; she would become, in the words of Sister Amadeus, "the long-time and expert head nurse for this unit." "The unit opened," Kate recalled, "with one head nurse, an assistant head nurse, eight registered nurses, four licensed practical nurses, and three aides for 24-hour coverage. Registerd nurses with experience as private duty nurses in neuro served as models for the staff. Working closely, the staff became like a family. For many years, staff turnover remained low. Sister Amadeus made certain that the unit was not without heavenly protection. Each bed had a cloth medal taped under the bed frame, out of sight.

"The intensive care unit involved close teamwork among all levels of caregiver . . . Working in the intensive care unit brought many challenges, both physical and emotional, to the nurses and physicians. Tears were not uncommon among the nurses. Empathy and compassion played an important part in the care and support of patients and relatives."

Ross H. Miller, M.D., a native of Oklahoma and graduate of the University of Oklahoma medical school, came to Mayo as a resident in 1950 and joined the staff in 1954. President of the Staff of Mayo Clinic in 1973, he was chair of the neurology department from 1975 to 1980. Dr. Spinner and colleagues note that Dr. Miller had "a unique clinical acumen for recognizing a patient with an underlying surgical lesion. He was a skilled, meticulous, but fast neurosurgeon, and he performed more than 4,000 operations for intracranial tumors."

Dr. Miller was also a self-effacing southern gentleman. Asked about Dr. McIlrath's comment, "Dr. Ross Miller made an outstanding contribution to the advancement of neurosurgery at Mayo," he deflected the recognition. "Every one of my colleagues was outstanding. Some of our surgeons, like Dr. Adson, Dr. MacCarty, and Dr. Sundt were notable for moving the department into new areas, but all of us worked together and learned from each other. Dr. MacCarty and I, for example, operated on the same day for many years in operating rooms adjacent to each other. During a surgery, if one of us had a question about a procedure or other matter, we would consult with the other. The opportunity to ask the opinion of a respected colleague was of vital importance in caring for our patients."

Thoralf M. Sundt II, M.D., followed Dr. Ross H. Miller as chair of the department from 1980 to 1992. Dr. Sundt, who was recruited by Dr. MacCarty, joined Mayo Clinic in 1969. "He quickly established himself," notes Spinner, as an innovative surgeon and investigator, particularly in cerebrovascular neurosurgery." Though many of Dr. Sundt's accomplishments are beyond the scope of this book, his great humanity had no boundaries. The striking tribute to Dr. Sundt, which follows, is also a tribute to his remarkable colleagues and all Mayo surgeons.

"Dr. Sundt was loved and respected by his patients. He was extremely kind and loyal to colleagues, residents, and nurses and was always accessible despite his heavy surgical and administrative schedule. Dr. Sundt was totally without pretense. Totally calm inside and outside the operating room, he had an uncommon resilience, discipline, and inner strength. Dr. Sundt's courageous battle against multiple myeloma was an inspiration to all who knew him; he lost his battle at home on the evening of September 9, 1992. To the last months of his life, he continued to display the attributes of kindness and courage. To many, he was the ultimate neurosurgeon, and his colleagues and residents felt privileged to have known, observed, and learned from him."

ENDNOTES

Page 155   Clagett OT: *General Surgery at the Mayo Clinic, 1900-1970*. Rochester, MN: self-published, 1980.

     Clapesattle H: *The Doctors Mayo*. Minneapolis: The University of Minnesota Press, 1941, pp 270, 273, 298-300, 358.

Page 156   Whelan E: *The Sisters' Story: Saint Marys Hospital—Mayo Clinic 1889-1939*. Rochester, MN: Mayo Foundation for Medical Education and Research, 2002, pp 80-81.

     Braasch WF: *Early Days in the Mayo Clinic*. Springfield, IL: Charles C Thomas, Publisher, 1969, p 69.

     Olmsted County Democrat September 22, 1905. Quoted in *Saint Marys Hospital News Bulletin* April 1964, p 1.

     History of Surgery at Mayo Clinic. [cited 2006 September 11]. Available from: http://www.mayoclinic.org/surgery/history/html.

     Mayo WJ: *The Future of the Clinic*. William J. Mayo Papers, Mayo Historical Suite.

     Whelan (pp 82, 90-91).

Page 157   Surgery: A History of Growth at Saint Marys. *Caring* Spring 1982, pp 2-4.

     Interview with Sister Paula Leopold, October 16, 2004.

     Dr. James T. Priestly Papers, Mayo Historical Suite.

Page 158   Interviews with Dr. Donald C. McIlrath, August 6, 2003 and February 22, 2006.

Pages 158-159   Clagett (pp 204-205).

Page 159   Clagett (pp 46-47).

     Interview with Dr. William "Bill" McConahey, October 19, 1998.

Pages 159-160   Interviews with Dr. Donald C. McIlrath, August 6, 2003 and February 22, 2006.

Page 160   **Clagett OT:** *World War II: General Surgery at the Mayo Clinic, 1900-1970*, **p 131.**

Celebrating 50 Years [videorecording]: The Development of Cardiopulmonary Bypass and Cardiac Surgery at Mayo Clinic: Presentations, Interviews and Photographs from May 12, 2005. Division of Cardiovascular Surgery, Mayo Clinic. **Rochester, MN: Mayo Clinic, 2005. Disc 1: Pairolero PC. Pioneers in Cardiology at Mayo Clinic.**

Pages 160-161   **Daly RC, Dearani JA, McGregor CGA, Mullany CJ, Orszulak TA, Puga FJ, Schaff HV, Sundt TM III, Zehr KJ: Fifty Years of Open Heart Surgery at the Mayo Clinic.** *Mayo Clin Proc* **2005;80:636-640.**

Page 161   **Kirklin JW: Open-Heart Surgery at the Mayo Clinic: The 25th Anniversary.** *Mayo Clin Proc* **1980;55:339-341.**

Celebrating 50 Years [videorecording], **Tape 1: Moffitt EA: Closing Remarks.**

Johnson V: *Mayo Clinic: Its Growth and Progress.* **Bloomington, MN: Voyageur Press, 1984, pp 92-97.**

Graner JL: *A History of the Department of Internal Medicine at the Mayo Clinic.* **Rochester, MN: Mayo Foundation for Medical Education and Research, 2002, p 261.**

Pages 161-162   Interview July 4, 2003 and letter of July 17, 2003 from Sister Merici Maher.

Pages 162-163   Interviews with Sister Carmen Sonnek, September 9, 2004 and August 31, 2006.

Page 163   Interview with Sister Cynthia Howe, August 9, 2005.

Saint Marys Annals, August 15, 1956.

Tells of 'Intensive Care' in Hospitals. *Saint Louis Post Dispatch* **April 15, 1959, p 2D.**

Pages 163-165   Interview with Sister Elizabeth Gillis, September 11, 2005.

Page 165   Interview with Sister Maeve Cashman (Marge Cashman Gallagher), September 26, 2006.

Pages 165-166   **Johnson V:** *Mayo Clinic: Its Growth and Progress*, **p 94.**

Page 166   Interview with Rosemary White, June 3, 2006.

Graner JL: *A History of the Department of Internal Medicine at the Mayo Clinic*, **p 262.**

Pages 166-167   **Spinner RJ, Al-Rodhan NRF, Piepgras DG: 100 Years of Neurological Surgery at the Mayo Clinic.** *Neurosurgery* 2001;49:438-446.

Page 167   **Klein Sister Amadeus: Neurological and Neurosurgical Nursing, Saint Marys Hospital, Rochester, Minnesota 1947-1960 (unpublished paper, not dated).**

Page 168   **Klein (unpublished paper).**

Whelan E: *The Sisters' Story: Saint Marys Hospital—Mayo Clinic 1889-1939*, **p 86.**

Interview with Sister Amadeus Klein, January 22, 2004.

Page 169   **Whelan (p 84).**

Interview with Dr. Collin MacCarty and son, Collin Stewart MacCarty, October 17, 1998.

Saint Marys Hospital Bulletin **May 1963, p 1.**

Page 170   **Michenfelder JD: Neuroanesthesia. In: Rehder K, Southorn P, Sessler A:** *Art to Science: Department of Anesthesiology at Mayo Clinic.* **Rochester, MN: Mayo Foundation for Medical Education and Research, 2000, pp 51-54.**

Towey C: Neurosurgical and Neurology Nursing in the Neuro ICU, 1958-1990 (unpublished paper, not dated).

Pages 170-171   **Spinner, Al-Rodhan, Piepgras (p 443).**

Page 171   Comments by Dr. Donald C. McIlrath, November 30, 2006.

Interview with Dr. Ross Miller, December 12, 2006.

Spinner, Al-Rodhan, Piepgras (p 445).

CHAPTER 9

The Faces of Change

The administrations of Sister Domitilla and Sister Generose are bookends for this story about Saint Marys Hospital. Sister Domitilla DuRocher, who succeeded Sister Mary Joseph Dempsey, led Saint Marys from 1939 to 1949. Sister Generose Gervais, the hospital's last Franciscan administrator, served from 1971 to 1981. The two Sisters shared a common French ancestry. Sister Domitilla was French on both sides of the family, Sister Generose, French and German. Their roots went deep on this continent—the Gervais family arrived in the 1600s while the DuRochers immigrated in the 1700s. Both families first came to French Canada and later to the United States. Perhaps a common Gallic heritage accounts for the Sisters' similar leadership qualities—high intelligence, quiet confidence, and fearless conviction.

The two Franciscans grew up in very different circumstances. In Monroe, Michigan the prosperous DuRochers raised a family of ten in a relatively privileged environment. The seven Gervais children, on the other hand, grew up on a hardscrabble farm in western Minnesota during the dust bowl era and the Great Depression. "Day after day," Sister Generose remembered, "the dust blew so hard we couldn't see across the front yard. The farm had no electricity, refrigeration, running water, or furnace. For fuel we burned corncobs from the barnyard in the kitchen stove. We raised corn, oats, barley, rye, and wheat—everything was done with horses. When I was 9, my father got his hand caught in a corn picker and lost all his fingers and most of the palm of his left hand. So my sister and I milked the cows and cleaned the muck in the barn and my brothers did all the chores. One entire summer I worked in the fields because we couldn't afford to hire a man to help. They were tough years," she said, "but we had a close family, a strong faith, and wonderful parents who taught us two important lessons—that we could aspire to higher goals and that every person deserves respect."

Taught by Rochester Franciscans in Currie, Minnesota, Sister Generose always wanted to be a Sister. She joined the congregation at 18, already an accomplished cook, baker, gardener and seamstress, thanks to her mother, an adult 4-H leader. Her first assignment was in Winona, Minnesota, teaching grade school. Within 2 years, she went to the University of Wisconsin at Stout to pursue a degree in Home Economics. Sister Generose presumed she would teach Home Economics until Mother Alcuin McCarthy, the general superior, told her that the congregation needed dietitians. "I don't know what a dietitian does," she responded, "but if you need one, I'm willing to try."

An openness to serve where needed combined with an extraordinary ability to master almost any assignment characterized Sister Generose. She was still a dietetic intern at Saint Marys Hospital in 1947 when Sister Domitilla asked her to direct the new practical nurse program. "I said I didn't know how I could be in charge when I wasn't a nurse." Reconsidering, Sister Domitilla appointed a nurse as director and named Sister Generose co-director. Later, Sister Generose served as assistant administrator to Sister Mary Brigh and as superior of the Saint Marys Hospital convent. In her capacity as superior she was an affirming, steadying presence for young Sisters, as noted in earlier chapters.

As associate administrator, Sister Generose worked closely with Sister Mary Brigh and chief engineer William O. Cribbs on major building projects. Sister Moira Tighe, friend and colleague over many years, commented, "Sister Generose could read blueprints as well as any architect. The men in Facilities Engineering liked to tell how she visualized exactly what was drawn on the print." "She was as comfortable with the complexity of blueprints as she was with canning fruit," noted another source. "Efficiency and attention to detail were her trademarks. She knew not only the square footage of every corner of the hospital, but how that space could best be utilized."

Plainspoken and direct, Sister Generose once confided, "If the need were there, I could probably do just about any job. But," she added, "I couldn't write a book." No matter, writers like colleague Marianne Hockema delighted in telling her story. "Sister was the consummate administrator. She had a passion for efficiency and an eye for detail. She was tireless . . . and I mean tireless. When I worked with Sister on a project we would work for

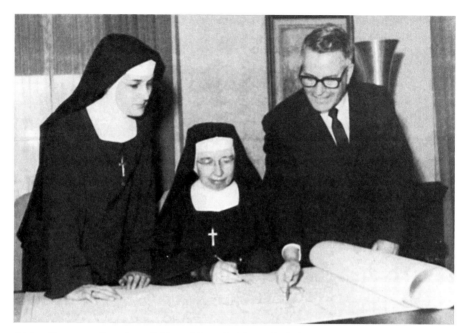

Sister Generose Gervais and Sister Mary Brigh worked closely with chief engineer, William O. Cribbs, on major hospital building projects. (From Saint Marys Hospital News Bulletin, Vol. XXII, no. 2, February 1963, p 1.)

several hours and I'd be exhausted. At this point, she was in her 60s and I was in my 40s. When I left for home at the end of the day, Sister would head for Mass, then a bite of supper and back to her office to pore over blue-prints, or to the kitchen to can thousands of jars of jam, jelly and pickles for the Sisters' annual bazaar. About midnight she'd head to the convent for a few hours of sleep before rising at 5 a.m."

Major building projects defined every decade between 1940 and 1980. Construction was a constant at Saint Marys—the Francis Building in the 1940s, the Domitilla Building in the 1950s, the Alfred Building in the 1960s and the Mary Brigh Building in the 1970s. As partners in the process, Sister administrators gained expertise from working with construction projects. Sister Domitilla used the experience she gained with the Francis Building when chair of the Domitilla Building Committee in the 1950s. Sister Mary Brigh, who worked closely with Sister Domitilla, took responsibility for the Alfred building in the 1960s with Sister Generose at her side. As hospital administrator in the 1970s, Sister Generose headed the 282 Project, which was dedicated on September 27, 1980.

The 282 Project added over 40 new operating rooms and a surgical suite that was as large as two football fields. The custom at Saint Marys was to officially name a new building at its dedication; having finished Project 281, engineers assigned a temporary name, "the 282 Project." The new structure also included 130 beds, two intensive care units, an enlarged emergency/trauma unit, and a new rehabilitation unit. According to *A Century of Caring: 1889-1989*, "The largest single hospital building project in Minnesota history," the project cost $55 million. To the delight of everyone assembled for the dedication, W. Eugene Mayberry, M.D., then chair of the Mayo Clinic Board of Governors, announced that the building would be named for Sister Mary Brigh Cassidy.

As early as the 1930s, Sister Domitilla initiated joint building committees comprised of Mayo and Saint Marys members. Her administrative successors followed the same practice. Joint committees gave Mayo and Saint Marys' colleagues the opportunity to accomplish a common goal that served the interests of both institutions. In the process, communication increased, mutual trust deepened, and a remarkable spirit of teamwork developed.

Gerald "Jerry" Mahoney, who served at Mayo from 1959 to 1996, was a member of several building committees. As administrative assistant, he worked on day-to-day operations with his counterparts at Saint Marys and Rochester Methodist Hospitals. Recalling his years at Mayo, Jerry's favorite word was "teamwork." "Teamwork made my job and just about everything else work well. It's the way we get things done at Mayo." His assignment as administrator for the hospital emergency rooms offered countless opportunities for teamwork. "When problems came up, the first thing I did was call one of the head nurses, Char Carey at Saint Marys or Irene Jensen at Methodist. They were terrific—together we could work out almost any problem. When you consider this kind of teamwork, it's pretty powerful. Underneath it, at least in my opinion, was our good working

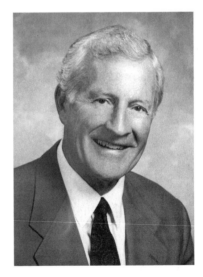

Gerald T. "Jerry" Mahoney, who served almost 40 years as Mayo administrator, currently chairs the Saint Marys Hospital Sponsorship Board. (From Mayo Clinic Archives.)

relationship, but even more important, each of us knew that the others shared the same goal. Above all, we wanted what was best for the patient."

Major construction at Saint Marys was prompted by Mayo's expanding clinical and surgical needs. In the early 1960s Mayo medical specialists approached Sister Mary Brigh about space for rapidly expanding research and clinical studies. Their request recalled a similar one that set a precedent 20 years earlier in 1941. At that time physicians asked Sister Domitilla about laboratory space for clinical studies in the new medical addition, later called the Francis Building. The Board of Governors concurred with their request. Sister Domitilla established a laboratory committee that worked with architects to include laboratories next to patient floors. With this initiative the Clinic would own the laboratories. Harry Harwick drew up a financial agreement, the first of its kind between the Clinic and Saint Marys Hospital. "In keeping with their partnership of 52 years, the two institutions sealed the agreement, not with a legal document, but with a handshake."

In 1967, the institutions made a similar, if more extensive, joint agreement on the Alfred Building. Approximately one-third of the ten-story building was dedicated to Mayo research and clinical studies. A lead article in a

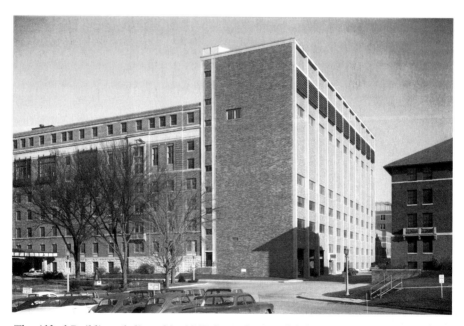

The Alfred Building, dedicated in 1967, housed research laboratories and clinical servic-es under one roof. (From A Century of Caring: 1889-1989. Rochester, MN: Saint Marys Hospital, 1998, p 99.)

1966 *Saint Marys News Bulletin* described the building and explained the reason for its name. "It is quite fitting that the new addition be named after Mother Alfred who pursued a dream to establish a hospital in which research could be realized."

The Gastroenterology Research Unit, hailed by the *Rochester Post-Bulletin* as "one of the most modern and sophisticated laboratories in the world," opened on June 21, 1967. Under the direction of William H. J. Summerskill, M.D., the unit had over 100 research projects and funding from the National Institutes of Health that included $2.5 million for research and $150,000 for research education.

Thirty-five years later, in an overview of the history of gastroenterology at Mayo, Philip W. Brown, Jr., M.D., made this comment. "The single most important event in our division proves to be the creation at Saint Marys Hospital of the GI Unit for Clinical Research. It was conceived by Hugh R. Butt [M.D.], modified by C. F. Code [M.D.], and brought to flower by its chief William H. J. Summerskill [M.D.] and his successors, Leslie J. Schoenfield [M.D., Ph.D], Sidney F. Phillips [M.D.], Alan F. Hofmann [M.D.], and Eugene P. DiMagno [M.D.]. Any GI consultant with an approved protocol can study a clinical condition with dedicated time and laboratory support."

The Alfred Building opened the same year that Mayo's Board of Governors

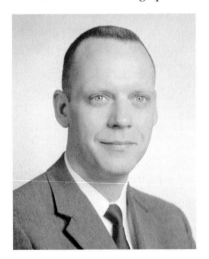

Richard Reitemeier, M.D., a nationally renowned physician, was the first chairman of the Department of Internal Medicine at Mayo Clinic. (From Mayo Clinic Archives.)

established a new Department of Internal Medicine. According to Mayo historian John Graner, an expanding technological medical environment was a major factor in their decision. "The Board of Governors decided it was time for an immediate change in Internal Medicine. A more traditional, hierarchical structure must be put in place, with a clear chain of command established." Prior to this time, medical services were divided into working groups called "sections," clusters of like subspecialists. Graner comments on this earlier arrangement that served the Clinic well. "Without a doubt the sectional concept was one of the factors most responsible for the solidarity of group practice at the Mayo Clinic. A non-threatening atmosphere . . . encouraged each staff member to perform at his or her maximum potential. Indeed, it made the great experiment of the first large private group practice of medicine and surgery a working reality."

The Mayo Board of Governors appointed gastroenterologist Richard Reitemeier, M.D., as the first chairman of the Department of Internal Medicine. Board of Governors Chairman, L. Emmerson Ward, M.D., commented on Dr. Reitemeier's appointment. "His abilities had shown themselves in a way which logically led him to become Chairman of the Department." During his career at the Clinic, Dr. Reitemeier "was one of the most prominent physicians in the country." The author of 121 articles and 21 abstracts and editorials, he was the recipient of numerous honors and awards and served on a wide range of national boards and committees. A native of Colorado, Dr. Reitemeier graduated from the University of Colorado medical school. After interning at Henry Ford Hospital in Detroit, Michigan, he came to Mayo as a resident in 1950 and joined the staff in 1954.

In his retirement, Dr. Reitemeier spoke about the enormous differences in clinical practice he found at Mayo. "We were peers and specialists. Unlike physicians throughout the country, careful to protect themselves and fearful of criticism, we were able to admit ignorance to each other, accept the fact we made mistakes, and support each other in this process. Our goal was 'to get the patient well, worry about the money later.' The Clinic supported us and generously provided medical care without charge to patients in need."

Dr. Reitemeier praised the dedication of staff as well as the Sisters and employees at every level of the organization. As a young resident he assisted renowned gastroenterologist J. Arnold Bargen, M.D., on Saint Marys' GI floor. "Most of these patients were unable to eat even small amounts of food—Dr. Bargen and head nurse Sister Gertrude Gaertner cared for them together. Sister Gertrude coaxed them to eat in every possible way, with lovely china and food she prepared herself. Dr. Bargen welcomed the opportunity to care for very sick patients." Later, Dr. Reitemeier wrote of his mentor's extraordinary effect on one of their patients.

"A young woman with severe ulcerative colitis of several years' duration was admitted to Saint Marys Hospital several days before Dr. Bargen was to begin his term as consultant in charge of such cases. She arrived emaciated, with a high fever, considerable abdominal pain, and the usual raging diarrhea. We did all that we could to make her comfortable, but her symptoms continued without change until the morning Dr. Bargen met her. He walked across the room and stood at the bedside of the patient, reaching out to grasp her right hand with his and placing his left hand on her forearm. Looking her straight in the eye, he said, 'I am so glad you have come! We are going to make you better!' He then went on with the usual interrogation of her history and a physical examination. However, we all noted that the very moment that he greeted her with that welcome assertion, she seemed to relax. As the day wore on, I was gratified and intrigued to watch all of her clinical signs improve. The fever abated, her diarrhea and abdominal pain quieted down, and indeed she did get better. I have always thought that the magic of his greeting was transferred to that woman through the warmth of his handshake and his evident honesty. He really did care about her."

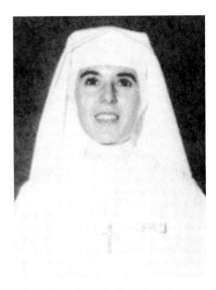

Sister Cashel Weiler's first assign-ment at Saint Marys was head nurse of the postoperative cardiac intensive care unit and cardiac unit. (From Saint Marys Hospital News Bulletin, Vol. XXVII, no. 8, August 1968.)

The cardiovascular division of internal medicine, like the GI division, opened expanded clinical research laboratories in the Alfred Building. Cardiologists W. Bruce Fye, M.D., and John A. Callahan, M.D., in an overview of the department, comment on con-tributing factors in cardiology's expanded role in the medical center. "Like cardiology throughout the United States, [it] was driven mainly by a combi-nation of technological advances, procedural innovations, and clinical demand. The whole process was fueled by the high prevalence of cardiovascular dis-ease, the rapid expansion of private health insurance after World War II, and the introduction of Medicare in 1966."

"The close and continuing collaboration of physicians, surgeons, scien-tists, and others from distinct but complementary disciplines," Graner noted in the last chapter of his history of the Department of Internal Medicine, "distinguished Mayo's heart program." Achievements in the develop-ment of the coronary care unit (CCU) in the 1960s and 1970s followed the remarkable collaborative standard set by open-heart surgery in the 1950s. Innovations that catalyzed the CCU movement, note Fye and Callahan, included "continuous ECG monitoring, the external defibrillator, the temporary transthoracic pacemaker, and cardiopulmonary resuscitation."

During this period, several Franciscan Sisters were directly involved with new coronary care initiatives. Sister Cashel Weiler's first assignment at Saint Marys was head nurse of the postoperative cardiac intensive care unit and cardiac unit. Sister Cashel, who succeeded Sister Colleen Waterman (Sister Darcy), commented on her predecessor's achievements. "Any success I had was predicated on the genius of Sister Colleen, who masterfully organized the unit before my arrival."

The unit had first-hand experience with the benefits of emerging technology. "A computerized method of regulating intravenous pumps was a wonderful contribution," recalled Sister Cashel. "We got that machine in 1967 and since there was only one, we had to decide which of our patients needed it most. For other patients needing IVs, nurses counted the drips to regulate dosage. Today, of course, automatic IV pumps are commonplace." In addition to the benefits of technology, Sister Cashel spoke of Sister Mary Brigh's good counsel. "As a young head nurse, she asked me to visit every patient daily. She said it would take just a few minutes to do an assessment of the patient's external condition. In that short time, I could judge if the patient was clean and comfortable and if anything was amiss in the room."

Sister Jennifer Corbett, who came to the unit in 1966, remembered how Sister Cashel interacted with staff. "Before leaving the unit at the end of the day, Sister Cashel sought out each person on the staff. She commented on their contributions that day and thanked them for it. She was sincere and consistent—it made a difference."

Many years later, asked about this practice, Sister Cashel, a little embarrassed, acknowledged the tribute. "Yes, that's what the staff says they remember about me. Just recently a nurse's aide told me what it meant to her." Sister Cashel went on to comment on one of Sister Jennifer's accomplishments, setting up classes for patients having heart surgery. "Before she joined our staff, our nurses went to wherever the patients were in the hospital and briefly informed them what to expect after heart surgery. Sister Jennifer planned and arranged for classes whereby the patients and relatives would come to class in the solarium on 3D. This saved time in the long run for the nurses because it consolidated the teaching. It also gave the relatives an opportunity to know one another before the surgery, and on the day of surgery to attend to, and to support each other. When the relatives arrived on the nursing floor, they were taken to the solarium to wait for word about their patients; they felt less alone seeing the familiar faces from the class the night before."

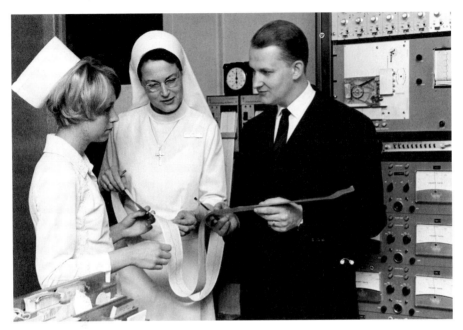

Sister Charlotte Dusbabek (center) confers with colleagues Tessie Ulrich (left) and Adolph H. Walser, M.D. (right). (From Mayovox, Vol. 21, no. 26, October 16, 1970, p 2.)

Historically, after postoperative cardiac care, the next stage in developing a dedicated CCU, note Fye and Callahan, "was the creation of a general medical intensive care unit at Saint Marys Hospital in 1964. Cardiologists John Callahan and James Broadbent [M.D.], the hospital administrator [Sister Mary Brigh], and members of the nursing service helped plan this unit that was designed and staffed to care for critically ill medical patients." Sister Charlotte Dusbabek (Sister Henry) served as head nurse of the first medical intensive care unit (ICU). "In a way," she said, "I was a pioneer. I had the opportunity to utilize the latest technology and techniques."

The experience of the medical ICU demonstrated the need for a dedicated cardiac intensive care unit. The unit opened in 1974; Sister Charlotte, as head nurse, recalled her experience in the ICUs. "Our excellent nursing staff worked as a team with the physicians who were equally dedicated. Caring for critically ill patients at the same time that we learned to use the new technology was a great challenge. Thankfully, even scientific innovation has its lighter side—I remember when a resident physician wrote in his orders that I was to stand in front of a particular patient's window and smile once a day!"

The momentum of change created by scientific and technological advances made an impact at Saint Marys beyond the operating rooms and ICUs. Major building projects, as noted earlier in this chapter, were a concrete example of the hospital's radically changing environment. Beyond bricks and mortar, the challenge of change has its own story in the evolution of three service departments, patient business services, pharmacy, and dietary.

As the new administrator in 1940, Sister Domitilla lost little time bringing change to hospital business practices. Informal structures of the past no longer met the hospital's needs. After establishing centralized purchasing and an accounting system, Sister Domitilla hired experienced laymen from outside the hospital to head them. When Sisters expressed concern that such changes threatened the spirit of Saint Marys, Sister Domitilla did not flinch. As noted in an earlier chapter, she called a meeting and stated her position. "Not any of us need to worry about the change in policy. It makes absolutely no difference to us if these men are Methodists, or Jews, or Hottentots. They were not secured to teach religion. They are experts in the things we want done and that is all that matters." As was their custom, Sisters complied out of dedication to the institution. Resistance to change, however, would continue to raise tensions in succeeding years.

Before the introduction of Medicare in 1966, business services experienced little change. Indeed, for over 10 years hospital publications carried the same description of the offices' purpose and function: "Saint Marys Hospital is not a business; it is a non-profit service institution. However, it is essential that the institution have an income and pay its bills if it is to meet the many needs of patient service. Hence the need of business offices and business policies. At Saint Marys, there are four offices directly concerned with business procedures, the cashiers' office, the collection office, the accounting offices, and the payroll office."

The cashiers' office, on the main floor of the Francis Building, was open every day of the week for patients to pay their bills. From 1949 to 1957 Sister JoAnne Lawson was night bookkeeper. A laywoman during these years, she worked alone from 7:00 in the evening until 7:00 the next morning. "My job was to keep the charges on each patient's account current," she explained. "Typically, the hospital had 850 patients. A private room was $3.75, a double $2.75, and wards were less. Color-coded vouchers with charges came from the departments. I used an NCR [National Cash Register] posting machine to update patient bills. Patient days ended at midnight. I had to balance every night and sometimes it took hours to reconcile a difference. In 1957,

I left Saint Marys to join the Franciscan congregation. After the novitiate, I went back to the hospital to work in the registration office and later became Registrar. I was delighted to work with patients directly and happy to renew friendships with employees and Sisters."

James "Jimmy" Drummond and a part-time secretary were responsible for all unpaid patient bills in the Collection Office. Patients were asked to pay one week in advance of their hospitalization. Mr. Drummond went to the floors as needed to help with payment arrangements and hospital insurance claims. Sister Corona Malis worked with Mr. Drummond when she arrived at Saint Marys in 1956. "He was a remarkable person," she said. "I suppose you could call him an 'unforgettable character' with his philosophical sayings and ready wit. He was also a gifted musician and gave concerts on the Clinic's carillon in Plummer Building for many years."

Sister Corona, whose first hospital assignment was the Accounting Office, served in that area for 38 years until she retired in 1994. During that time, she shared an office with friend and mentor, Sister Millicent Kuechenmeister, the hospital's treasurer. Both tireless workers, they were in the office literally day and night. Asked about her long hours, Sister Corona responded, "That's what we all did. In those years, there were just a few of us in the offices. Sister Aquila [Myers], for example, was a teacher who came to help out one summer and stayed for 28 years. She did her job quietly with great dedication. When she retired, they replaced her with seven people!

Other Sisters were much like her, Sister Rita Rishavy, Sister Marcellita Dempsey, and Sister Petrine DeSplinter among them. Saint Marys was our hospital, our responsibility, and we had an important mission— to serve patients. Working in the business offices was our way of serving patients, of doing God's work."

Lively and vivacious, Sister Corona enjoyed her work for its variety of tasks and the opportunity to interact with people. "Sister Corona touches

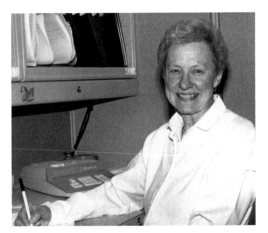

Sister Corona Malis, Patient Counselor in the Accounting Office, served in that department for 38 years. (From Caring, Summer 1989, p 5. Rochester, MN: Saint Marys Hospital.)

others' lives," wrote a colleague, "with her own joy and warmth." As Patient Counselor, like James Drummond, she helped patients make payment arrangements for their hospital bills. "We didn't harass patients for payment and no one was turned away from the hospital," she said emphatically. "We wrote off millions of dollars—some people simply couldn't pay their bills."

Sister Corona prepared a monthly accounting report for Administration. "We received regular reports from most of the offices and departments," recalled executive secretary Sister Lauren Weinandt. "I helped Sister Mary Brigh, and later Sister Generose, prepare weekly, monthly, and annual administrative reports." Sister Lauren used her trusted manual typewriter for all business, including multicolumn financial reports, a Herculean task. Sister Generose, who preferred to work with financial data by hand, was a genius in reading reports. With painstaking attention, she checked all statistical reports against her own figures and relentlessly pursued any discrepancies.

Sister Mary Brigh began the practice of inviting employees to a presentation on the hospital's annual report. The session, which lasted an hour, concluded with refreshments. "Sister Mary Brigh could make the figures dance," remembered Sister Lauren. Sister Generose, who continued the tradition, offered sessions at a variety of times to include all employees who wished to attend. These efforts bore fruit—a more informed and invested staff. Of course, there were always exceptions. Sister Moira recalled that one employee, typically not interested in reports, attended several sessions. When asked about this new interest, the employee responded. "Well, Sister, I suppose the reports were okay. But what I really liked were the desserts they served this year."

Sister Dorothy Verkuilen (Sister Armand), new to Saint Marys in 1959, became the first coordinator for Patient Business Services. She coordinated six

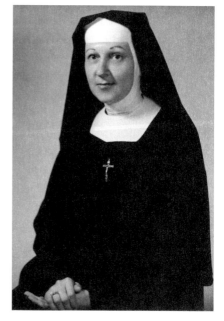

Sister Lauren Weinandt, administrative assistant to the hospital administrator, had wide and varied responsibilities. (Courtesy of Sister Lauren Weinandt.)

areas, the Information Desk, Registration, Cashiers, Credit Office, Telephone Office, and Patient Escorts. Her personal gifts, along with business experience prior to entering the congregation, served her well in the new position. "I enjoyed learning new tasks and liked to get to the bottom of things," she said. "I could see some changes would be helpful, but consulted with the staff first. Comments and suggestions from these dedicated, experienced employees were invaluable."

In the 1960s and 1970s, three young men came to work at Saint Marys, Larry D. Albrecht, Robert "Bob" Craven, and Thomas "Tom" Pool. Larry, from rural Rochester, was 17 and just out of high school when he started at the hospital in 1964. Tom Pool and Bob Craven, both in their 20s, arrived in the 1970s. Bob, who served as the hospital's first comptroller, originally came from Minneapolis. Tom, from west-central Illinois, assisted with Saint Marys' first computer. None of them were Catholic and only Tom had worked with Sisters. Saint Marys Hospital promised to be a great adventure.

Several senior Sisters reported, at least formally, to Bob Craven as comptroller; Sister Millicent, the hospital's treasurer, was one of them. "Sister Millicent, while very capable, was a quiet, self-effacing person and difficult to know," Bob recalled. "I persisted and got to know a wonderful woman who cared deeply about our patients and employees. Sister Millicent and Sister Mary Brigh taught me some important lessons. One of them was how to handle errors. I was impressed that the Sisters looked inward for solutions, not outward. If something went wrong, they didn't blame anyone. Instead, they studied the problem, and then asked themselves, 'What went wrong? How can we improve?' I remember an instance when a patient refused to pay a bill because he thought we overcharged him. Sister Mary Brigh carefully examined all the charges. 'The bill is accurate and fair,' she concluded. 'We can't change the charges. But if the patient isn't able to pay the bill, that's another matter. We can handle that in a different way.'"

"When I began in the business offices," said Larry Albrecht, "I was fortunate to work for Sister Dorothy. She assigned me to almost every office. I worked in registration, in accounting, filled in for the night bookkeeper, and served as a patient escort. I got to know the hospital and the Sisters. As an escort, I picked up patients when they were discharged from the floors and took them in wheel chairs to the hospital door. I remember that Sister Gloria Hoffman and Sister Cashel Weiler never let a patient leave their floors without saying goodbye. They'd get right down on the patient's eye level to answer questions and offer reassurance.

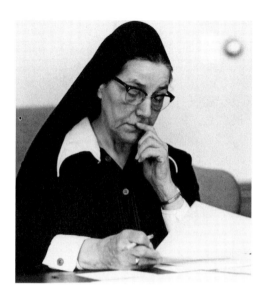

The hospital's highly capable treasurer, Sister Millicent Kuechenmeister, worked "literally day and night." (From Saint Marys Hospital Archives.)

"Saint Marys first impressed me as rather dark and old-fashioned looking. The hospital used only incandescent bulbs and the halls were dim at night. After fluorescent lights were installed, Saint Marys took on a different look, almost like it stepped into the modern age. In those years the hospital was not so much of a business—it was more like a family. On weekends, when we had a skeleton crew, everyone pitched in. Sister Millicent and Sister Generose took their turns at the information desk as did other Sisters. If the plumbing didn't work in one of the bathrooms, Sister Lucas [Chavez] came from the convent to take care of the problem."

In 1971, Saint Marys took a significant step into the modern age with the installation of a new computer system. With 33 nursing stations, 4 pharmacies, and over 1,000 beds, the hospital required a more efficient system for communicating and processing information. About 5 years earlier, Sister Florence Zweber (Sister Aquinette), previously a nursing administrator, was appointed Assistant Administrator for Fiscal Affairs and Systems Management. Tall, slender, and immaculately dressed, she seemed to glide down the hospital's halls. Sister Florence, who brought intelligence, high energy, and purpose to every assignment, concentrated on innovative ideas. Larry Albrecht, who currently serves in Mayo's Systems department, remembered her interest in the hospital as a system. "She'd ask questions like, 'What steps do you use to get from here to there? How do people communicate patient information within their departments? How do they communicate patient information to other departments?'"

At Sister Florence's direction, Saint Marys purchased a total information and communications system called "Medelco." One of her administrative colleagues wryly observed, "Sister Florence was inclined to take action and ask forgiveness later." Not surprisingly, such a unilateral decision was

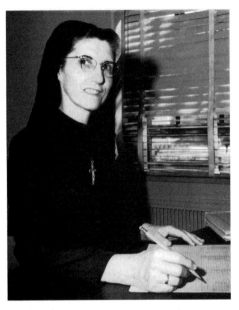

Assistant Administrator for Fiscal Affairs and Systems Management, Sister Florence Zweber introduced computers to Saint Marys Hospital. (From Saint Marys Hospital Archives.)

not appreciated by some of her peers. Undaunted, Sister Florence created a new systems department to expedite Medelco operations and coordinate interdepartmental changes. Ultimately, Medelco provided trained personnel and computer terminals throughout the hospital.

Tom Pool, who first came to Saint Marys as an employee of Medelco, assisted with the computer's installation and monitored initial operations. "Sister Florence," said Tom, "single-handedly brought Medelco to Saint Marys. She assessed the hospital's current and future needs, studied the options, and made the decision to use Medelco. Amazingly, in spite of criticism and misunderstandings, she managed to pull it off. Saint Marys Hospital was one of the first hospitals in the country to have a comprehensive computer system on the level of Medelco."

As a Medelco employee, Tom was impressed by Saint Marys' commitment to excellence and the staff's dedication to patients. When the hospital offered him a position in the systems department, he was happy to accept. The decision was a fortunate one in many respects; chiefly, it gave Tom the opportunity to meet and marry a lovely young Saint Marys' employee, Jean Tlougan. Introduced to the hospital when she became a candy striper, Jean has served in a variety of areas, currently with Mayo's Department of Human Resources.

"The new Systems Department," said Tom, "consisted of four people and two of them were Franciscans." Sister Dorothy Verkuilen applied her considerable skills on day-to-day operations and tackled a variety of new challenges. Sister Manette Tisdale became a systems analyst with the informal title of "problem solver." Sister Manette helped departments incorporate Medelco through hands-on instruction and written manuals. "She gave 110% to her job," commented Tom Pool. Sister Manette's wit, entertaining comments, and thoughtful ways made her a great favorite among peers and patients alike. Observing her interactions with patients in elevators, offices, and hallways, a visitor commented, "You're the hospital's 'hallway ambassador.'" Sister Manette responded, "If I see a person walking alone or crying I stop and talk or give comfort. I make a point of this because there is so much good that can be done by giving a little to people in need."

The pharmacy department, directed by Sister Kathleen Van Groll (Sister Torello), was one of the first departments to incorporate Medelco. Sister Kathleen assigned the project to Louise Kortz, Pharm.D., an experienced, highly competent pharmacist. "It was a difficult process, but the job needed to be done." said Louise. "I started by putting numbers on every drug in the department. With help from Sister Manette and working closely with [the Department of] Nursing, we incorporated pharmacy into the Medelco system."

Appointed pharmacy director in the mid 1960s, Sister Kathleen succeeded Sister Quentin McShane, who held the position for almost 25 years. Sister Quentin, a respected director, was a genteel, outgoing woman with an engaging sense of humor. Sister Kathleen, tall and distinguished looking, had a reserved, businesslike demeanor that contrasted with the more light-hearted Sister Quentin. Both women assumed the director position at a time of significant change in the profession. Pharmaceutical advances brought about by World War II, penicillin and sulfa among them, had a major impact when Sister Quentin began in the early 1940s. Twenty years later, the dramatic increase in drugs and their complex interactions brought the profession to a new era. "The pharmacist has evolved," noted a hospital publication, "into a professional who must understand the role of drugs in any given disease and be able to communicate that understanding to other health professionals."

Sister Kathleen's inquisitive mind and organizational skills served her well as she guided the department in new directions. "Sister Kathleen was open to ideas and they didn't have to be her own," commented a group of retired pharmacists. "If the idea seemed reasonable, she never told us we couldn't try something. But gone were the days when we made window washing solution in the back room, to say nothing of black shoe polish and deodorant for the Sisters!" Mayo accountant Robert "Bob" Perez spoke about his first job at Saint Marys in the pharmacy. "Sister Kathleen hired me—I was a pharmacy tech before they named the job and created a training program. She was a wonderful woman and I'll always be grateful for her personal interest and help. Sister Kathleen was patient and understanding, but she knew how to straighten me out, too," said Bob with a smile. "As the only girl among five brothers, I guess she'd had some experience in that area."

About the same time that Sister Kathleen became pharmacy director, Sister Florence was appointed Assistant Administrator for Fiscal Affairs and Systems Management. The two women took the lead on several important projects in the pharmacy department, including the creation of decentralized pharmacies. At the opening of the surgical pharmacy in 1972, Sister Kathleen addressed its purpose. "The basic advantage of the decentralized pharmacy is its proximity to the patient care area." She went on to explain pharmacy's new practice of preparing and delivering medications in unit doses to nursing floors. "Centralized unit-dose dispensing," Sister Kathleen attested, "will cut the nurse's time spent preparing and dispensing medication by 50 to 75%."

To meet the needs of the expanding department, Sister Kathleen hired Mick Hunt as assistant director in 1972. A brilliant young pharmacist, Mick Hunt introduced training in the preparation and delivery of IVs as well as unit doses of medications. Hunt created the pharmacy tech position and accompanying training program to provide skilled personnel for the preparation and distribution of IVs and unit doses. Hunt's creation of the pharmacy tech

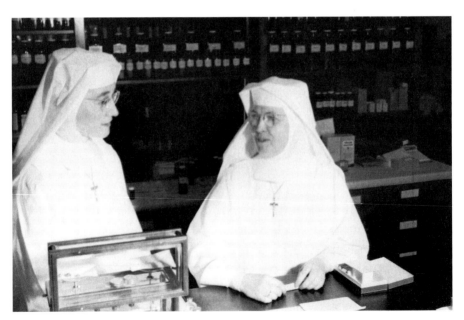

Two capable Franciscans led the pharmacy department: Sister Quentin McShane (right), followed by Sister Kathleen Van Groll (left). (From Saint Marys Hospital Archives.)

program bore fruit beyond the pharmacy department. Kate Towey, head nurse in the neurologic ICU for many years, commented on this welcome change. "Pharmacy techs delivered medications and made a daily check of narcotics, replacing them as needed. They also delivered and assisted with IVs. These services were of great help to our unit personnel."

Retired pharmacy education coordinator, Joseph "Joe" Kostick, commented on Mick Hunt's contributions to the department. "Mick initiated an educational component in pharmacy that changed the way we worked. He established the pharmacy residency program and promoted in-service staff education. Hunt's pharmacy tech program taught techs the skills to do tasks formerly handled by pharmacists. At a time of changing roles for pharmacists, this assistance was invaluable. Pharmacists were now freed to meet a range of new expectations—to become more involved with clinical issues and more knowledgeable about the growing number of drugs. Increasingly, pharmacists became recognized leaders in their specialty, consulted by physicians and other members of the medical team."

Unlike pharmacy, the dietary department was not quick to adopt computer technology. Existing services, such as the pneumatic tube system, initially met their interdepartmental communication needs. Dietary's roots went back to the hospital's beginnings, when one of its founders, Sister Fidelis Cashion, arrived "to take care of the cuisine." The dietary department took an expanded role when diet therapy became a major component of medical treatment. Russell M. Wilder, M.D., a key person in developing nutrition services at Mayo Clinic, moved to Saint Marys, accompanied by Daisy Ellithorpe, Rochester's first dietitian. The medical department conducted extensive clinical investigations using controlled food intake for diseases including diabetes mellitus, nephritis, osteoporosis, arthritis, and Addison's disease. Commenting on the contribution of these studies, Dr. Wilder noted, "It could be said that clinical investigation at Saint Marys stimulated the rapid development of dietetics."

One of dietetics' pioneer leaders, Florence Hazel Smith, headed dietetic services at Saint Marys. Sisters Joseph and Domitilla, however, believed that a Sister with appropriate educational preparation should eventually head the department. Sister Victor Fromm, who later called herself "a renegade nurse," recalled how she had just graduated from Saint Marys School of Nursing "when Sister Domitilla persuaded me to go into dietetics." When Florence Smith left Saint Marys, Sister Victor took her place in 1927 and became a renowned leader in her field.

As the reputation of the department grew, an increasing number of students, national and international, asked to study at Saint Marys. European fellows of the Rockefeller Foundation came from England, Poland, and Yugoslavia for postgraduate study in the department. In response to these numerous applications, Sister Victor organized an internship program in dietetics in 1930 with approval from the American Dietetics Association. Interns received graduate credit for academic preparation and hands-on experience in food service administration and clinical dietetics. In addition, they were introduced to community nutrition and metabolic research. The acclaimed internship program continues to the present day.

With Sister Victor's resignation in 1970, Sister Moira Tighe became director of the 300-employee department. Sister Moira's career in dietary, which spanned 44 years, included experience in every area of the department. Dietary administration had unique challenges. Employees assigned to the preparation and distribution of meals for patients and staff worked a split shift, 7 a.m. to 1:30 p.m., and then from 4 p.m. to 7 p.m. In addition, due to the diversity of jobs within the department, employees represented a wide array of abilities and educational backgrounds from 8th grade graduates to Ph.D.s. Known for her firm and fair leadership, along with a droll sense of humor, Sister Moira was clearly up to the task.

The dietetic internship program brought Bernadette Novack (Sister Richard) to Saint Marys in 1959 from her home in Edina, Minnesota. Her studies in food service administration would have far-reaching consequences. After her internship, Sister Bernadette worked at Saint Marys for about a year before she chose to enter the Rochester Franciscans. Following the novitiate, she returned to Saint Marys and the dietary department. "I liked living in the convent and getting to know the Sisters. There were 120 of us when I arrived in 1963."

Sister Bernadette, who used the skills she learned as an intern, taught new interns menu planning, food purchasing and cost control, quantity food preparation and service, and employee management. Bernadette enjoyed the interaction with employees and the hands-on experience of learning from experts in their fields like Harry Benson, supervisor of the meat shop for 50 years and "the ice cream lady," Clara Blackburn. "Clara made all the ice cream, 120 gallons of the mix, for the hospital's Ice Cream Socials. With help from employees in the bakery Sister Barnabas Schroeder made her famous doughnuts and the bakery produced several hundred dozen sugar cookies. As staff waited in long lines, the sun, shining on the sugar cookies, produced the aroma of fresh baked cookies right out of the oven."

Sister Rose Gillespie joined Sister Bernadette as an administrative dietitian in 1969 when she transferred to the Rochester Franciscans from another religious congregation. Sister Rose, a registered dietitian, also brought credentials and experience in educational administration. Reflecting on her preference for health care over education, she said, "I always felt health care put my life in perspective. It taught me that life was larger than I was and made me thankful for my health and for opportunities to serve. To me the Sisters who served in the kitchen reflected those values."

The Sisters in the kitchen, like their peers in the laundry and housekeeping, were essential to the hospital. Almost all them came to their assignments as young women right out of the novitiate, and stayed for 40, 50, even 60 years. Though they worked behind the scenes, they were as committed to serving patients as any Sister in surgery or on a nursing floor. Further, they recognized the importance of their contribution and took great pride in the accomplishments of Saint Marys Hospital and Mayo Clinic.

In her appointment as in-service dietary coordinator, Sister Rose used both her educational background and dietetics training. The classes gave her an opportunity to know dietary's 300 employees—she made it a practice to call each person by name. Now retired, Sister Rose spoke about her experience in dietary. "I was always impressed with the dedication of staff members. Employees would call when a bad snowstorm was on the way to ask for sleeping rooms at the hospital so they wouldn't miss their shift. To put forth that extra effort showed how much they cared about their work and each other."

This chapter, focusing on the faces of change created by scientific and technical advances, describes the effects on a wide diversity of hospital areas. However, from ICUs to business offices and pots and pans, staff and employees shared a common commitment. "The capstone of this commitment," wrote Larry Albrecht "is joy in fulfilling the mission. Shared by many of the people I've talked with (but not all), it was much more than a paycheck. Those who didn't relate directly to patients 'helped to hold the place together' so that others could give the best patient care. Our mission went above physician demands and supervisors' expectations. We extended ourselves, so that everyone who entered our doors, patient and family alike, experienced the best we all had to give."

ENDNOTES

Page 175 — Interviews with Sister Generose Gervais, January 28, 2000 and February 25, 2005.

Pages 175-176 — Presentation by Sister Ellen Whelan, Sponsorship Retreat, January 15, 2002.

Page 176 — Interview with Sister Generose Gervais, March 5, 2005.

Interview with Sister Moira Tighe, October 4, 2005.

Pages 176-177 — **Hockema M: *The Franciscan Five* (unpublished paper, Saint Marys Hospital Archives), p 39.**

Pages 177-178 — *A Century of Caring: 1889-1989.* **Rochester, MN: Saint Marys Hospital, 1988, p 100.**

Page 178 — Interview with Gerald T. Mahoney, November 3, 2006.

Page 179 — **Whelan E: *The Sisters' Story, Part Two: Saint Marys Hospital—Mayo Clinic, 1939-1980.* Rochester, MN: Mayo Foundation for Medical Education and Research, 2007, Chapter 2, pp 32-34.**

Pages 179-180 — *Saint Marys Hospital News Bulletin* **August-September, 1966.**

Page 180 — **Rochester Post-Bulletin quotes in the *Saint Marys Hospital News Bulletin* November 1967.**

Brown P Jr: The Division of Gastroenterology. In: *A History of the Department of Internal Medicine at the Mayo Clinic.* Edited by JL Graner. Rochester, MN: Mayo Foundation for Medical Education and Research, 2002, p 238.

Pages 180-181 — **Graner (pp 30-31).**

Page 181 — Interview with Dr. Richard Reitemeier, August 5, 2003.

Pages 181-182 — **Manning PR, DeBakey L: *Medicine: Preserving the Passion.* New York: Springer-Verlag, 1987, p 200.**

Caring **Summer 1989, p 14.**

Page 182   **Fye WB, Callahan JA: The Division of Cardiovascular Diseases. In:** *A History of the Department of Internal Medicine at the Mayo Clinic.* **Edited by JL Graner, p 262.**

Interviews with Sister Cashel Weiler, May 31, 2006 and September 20, 2006.

Page 183   Interview with Sister Jennifer Corbett, June 29, 2005.

Pages 183-184   **Fye WB, Callahan JA (pp 263-264).**

Page 184   Interview with Sister Charlotte Dusbabek, February 3, 2006.

Page 185   **Whelan E:** *The Sisters' Story, Part Two: Saint Marys Hospital—Mayo Clinic, 1939-1980,* **Chapter 3, p 45.**

Saint Marys Hospital News Bulletin **August 1949.**

Saint Marys Hospital News Bulletin **January 1959.**

Pages 185-186   Interviews with Sister JoAnne Lawson, August 3, 2003 and June 30, 2004.

Pages 186-187   Interview with Sister Corona Malis, September 13, 2005.

Page 187   Interviews with Sister Lauren Weinandt, May 15, 2006 and July 24, 2006.

Interview with Sister Moira Tighe, December 1, 2006.

Pages 187-188   Interview with Sister Dorothy Verkuilen, December 4, 2005.

Page 188   Interview with Robert Craven, November 10, 2006.

Pages 188-189   Interview with Larry Albrecht, November 24, 2006.

Page 189   Interview with Roger Wells, February 9, 2006.

Page 190   Interviews with Thomas Pool, November 29, 2006, December 13, 2006, and January 4, 2007.

Pages 190-191   *Caring* **Summer 1989, p 17.**

Page 191   Interview with Louise Kortz, December 14, 2006.

Caring **Spring 1984, p 3.**

Group Pharmacy Interview with Beverly Allen, Joseph P. Kostick, Naomi Stanek, and Richard J. Streit, September 21, 2005.

Interview with Robert Perez, November 27, 2006.

Page 192   *Saint Marys Hospital News Bulletin* **May 1972.**

Towey C: *Neurosurgical and Neurology Nursing in the Neuro ICU, 1958-1990* (unpublished paper, not dated, Saint Marys Hospital Archives).

Page 193   Interview with Joseph Kostick, December 16, 2006.

Whelan E: *The Sisters' Story: Saint Marys Hospital—Mayo Clinic 1889-1939.* Rochester, MN: Mayo Foundation for Medical Education and Research, 2002, pp 128, 129.

Pages 193-194   **Whelan (pp 130, 131).**

Page 194   *Caring* **Summer 1989, p 3.**

Caring **Summer 1989, p 16.**

Interviews with Sister Bernadette Novack, August 3, 2005 and December 10, 2006.

Novack B: *History Tidbits for Saint Marys Hospital Dietetics Department* (unpublished paper, Saint Marys Hospital Archives).

Page 195   **Whelan (p 132).**

Interviews with Sister Rose Gillespie, September 12, 2005 and December 8, 2006.

Letter from Larry Albrecht, November 27, 2006.

CHAPTER 10

Forging a Franciscan Legacy

The 1960s held great promise. John Fitzgerald Kennedy, whose presidential inauguration opened the decade, challenged a new generation of Americans to fight tyranny, poverty, and disease. "To those peoples in the huts and villages of half the globe struggling to break the bonds of mass misery," he proclaimed, "we pledge our best efforts to help them help themselves." Within months, President Kennedy created the Peace Corps with the mandate "to promote world peace and friendship." Inspired by idealism and generosity, Americans responded in striking numbers. By 1963, 7,000 Peace Corps volunteers served in 44 countries from Afghanistan to Uruguay.

In 1962, the world watched as 2,500 men, the collective leadership of the Roman Catholic Church, marched to St. Peter's Basilica and opened the Second Vatican Council. "So rare are Councils," noted *Time* magazine, "there have been only 20 in nearly 2,000 years of Christian history." The Council was the inspiration of Pope John XXIII, *Time's* Man of the Year: "John's historic mission is fired by a desire to endow the Christian faithful with 'a new Pentecost,' a new spirit. It is aimed not only at bringing the mother church of Christendom into closer touch with the modern world, but at ending the division that has dissipated the Christian message for four centuries."

In his opening message, Pope John asked church leaders to face new challenges with a pastoral spirit. "We want to fix a steady gaze on those who still lack the opportune help to achieve a way of life worthy of human beings. As we undertake our work, therefore, we would emphasize whatever concerns the dignity of man, whatever contributes to the community

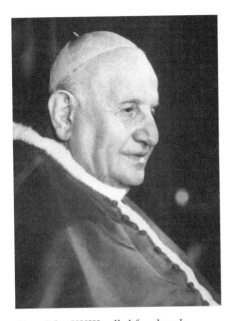

Pope John XXIII called for church reform and renewal in the Second Vatican Council (1962-1965). (From Walsh M: An Illustrated History of the Popes: Saint Peter to John Paul II. New York: St. Martin's Press, 1980, p 218.)

of peoples." Though John XXIII called for renewal, powerful prelates within the Curia, the Vatican bureaucracy, opposed change. "Curialists," as they were called, attempted to block reform at every turn. Nevertheless, notes historian Christopher M. Bellito, "Almost from the start of the council a spirit of independence upset the curialists' stalling maneuvers. It was a global meeting, full of young churches; while Europeans made up of 33% of those in attendance, 35% came from North and South America, 10% each from Africa and Asia.

"Three innovations would lead to reform: a commission for the laity . . . a secretariat to promote Christian unity . . . and non-curial diocesan bishops and theologians were appointed to the commissions. These experts (*periti*, to use the familiar Latin word) included some theologians whose work had been suspected and even censured in earlier decades. Their ideas soon overcame the curialists' program and their talks during the four autumn sessions (1962-1965) drew overflow crowds of bishops eager to update their own theological training. Each fall during the early sixties, Rome turned into one big seminar."

The Sisters at Saint Marys Hospital, like most Americans, looked to the 1960s with high hopes. President Kennedy's creation of a Peace Corps resonated with their idealism and commitment to the underprivileged. John XXIII's call for a council of renewal promised hope for the church. Church renewal offered hope that religious orders could change outmoded rules to fit the present times. The volatile 1960s indeed changed institutions and attitudes. A new generation questioned societal standards, not the least of these the position of women in society. Within the decade, congregational renewal became a reality. The momentum and scope of change, however, created unforeseen consequences for Saint Marys Hospital. This chapter tells the Sisters' story of Saint Marys Hospital within the context of the renewal whose roots, changes, and outcomes made a lasting impact.

Religious life in 1965 had not changed appreciably since 529AD, when Benedict of Nursia founded Western monasticism at Monte Cassino. Uniformity and obedience were behavioral ideals for a lifestyle that centered on communal prayer, meditative silence, and a cloistered environment. "Sisters arose at the same time, prayed and ate together, always in assigned places and often in silence. Permission from superiors was required for most activities, especially leaving the convent, making phone calls and sending letters and receiving visitors. The vow of obedience was strictly followed." Under the vow of obedience, Sisters were assigned to Saint Marys by the congregational superior. At Saint Marys, the hospital administrator assigned professional responsibilities. An exception occurred in the mid 1960s. When the congregation established foundations in Latin America, Sisters were invited to volunteer for these assignments.

Early in the 1960s Pope John asked American religious orders to help the peoples of Latin America; he urged every congregation to dedicate 10% of their membership to this effort. The response from Rochester Franciscans came quickly. The congregation's general superior, Mother Callista Hynes, accompanied by Sister Mary Brigh, made a 2-week tour of educational and medical facilities in Colombia, Panama, Guatemala, and Mexico. Upon return, Mother Callista announced that five Sisters would go to Bogota, Colombia, in September of 1962, "to establish a school for upper-middle class girls on the high school level." "We hope," said Mother Callista, "our school in Bogota will provide young women who will become future teachers, dietitians, nurses, and leaders in the years to come." To the Colombians' delight and gratitude, the Sisters established Colegio Santa Francisco Romana in February 1963. The Colegio gave Sisters a base to reach out to the poor. Typically, after a day at school, they went to the nearby barrio to serve the poor who lived there.

Prior to her 2006 election as president of the Sisters of Saint Francis, Sister Tierney Trueman served 31 years in Bogota as Coordinator of the Franciscan Mission in Colombia. Sister Tierney commented on the origin of Franciscan health care services during her years in Bogota: "In the early 1980s, several graduates of the Colegio who were studying medicine began to offer medical care to the poor of the area. They opened the *Dispensario Santa Francisca Romana*, a drop-in clinic on the grounds of the *Colegio*." "Today," she continued, "the *Dispensario* offers the services of over 30

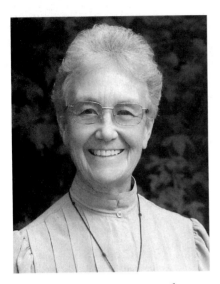

Sister Tierney Trueman currently serves as president of the Sisters of Saint Francis, Rochester, Minnesota. (From Assisi Heights Archives.)

medical specialists. In addition, senior medical, dental, nursing, and physical therapy students from four universities provide on-site clinical care as well as home care for patients unable to visit the clinic."

In 1963, with congregational approval, Franciscans responded to health care needs in Bogota. At the invitation of Universidad Javeriana, the Jesuit university, three Sisters from Saint Marys Hospital entered the nursing field in Latin America, Sister Jean Schulte (Sister Lea), assistant director of the College of Saint Teresa nursing program, along with nursing supervisors, Sister Seamus (Carol McKenna), and Sister Maeve (Marge Cashman Gallagher).

Appointed as the university's first Dean of Nursing, Sister Jean established a baccalaureate nursing program and phased out the existing 3-year program. Sister Maeve directed nursing service at the university's Hospital de San Ignacio, and Sister Seamus supervised pediatrics and the emergency room.

Sister Jean, who served as dean from 1963 to 1968, recalled her first impressions. "The lack of qualified faculty, teaching resources, and funds was immediately apparent. I met with the Kellogg Foundation when they conducted a site visit in the university's medical school. We applied to Kellogg and were fortunate to receive a $300,000 grant. With grant moneys we sent our best Colombian candidate to Boston College for a nursing degree. In the meantime, I worked with Colombian nurses to incorporate the baccalaureate program and phase out the three-year program. We brought nursing consultants to Bogota from the States. Irene Beland from Wayne State University was excellent, as were Jean Brennan and Dorothy Titt from the University of Minnesota. Many institutions helped us in a variety of ways. As a graduate of the University of Minnesota's Masters Program in Nursing, I was particularly grateful to the Department of Nursing for their generous support and professional assistance.

"From the onset, I had specific goals in mind. For one, I wanted to base our program on the core nursing principle I learned at Saint Marys Hospital:

'The patient is our central focus.' Another goal was inspired by a book I read before I went to Bogota, *The Nun in the World*. The author, Cardinal Joseph Suenens, urged missionaries to respect and honor the people in the countries they served. My goal was to give native Colombians the tools they needed to lead the program themselves. And that's what happened—I worked myself out of a job!" Sister Jean's picture now hangs in the School of Nursing at Universidad Javeriana. Asked about the university's tributes to her over the years, she comment-

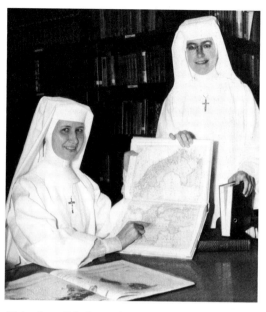

Sister Jean Schulte and Sister Seamus McKenna (Carol McKenna) responded to Pope John XXIII's call to serve health care needs in Latin America. (From Saint Marys Hospital Archives.)

ed, "Colombians are unusually gracious people. I believe they appreciated the high standard of nursing I brought to the program."

In 1963, Rochester Franciscans and other American Sisters established a ministry in Peru to help native Sisters raise their level of education. They came at the invitation of Peru's papal representative Archbishop Romulo Carbone. The Sisters were members of the Sister Formation movement, founded some 10 years earlier to promote the spiritual, professional, and intellectual formation of young Sisters. The Franciscans' training in Spanish and their professional preparation served them well. An instructor at the College of Saint Teresa, Sister Gretchen Berg, who headed the project, had recently received her Ph.D. in English Literature from the Catholic University of America. Sister Romana Walch, chair of Saint Teresa's education depart-ment, made a key contribution, as did Sister Consuelo (Marguerite) Chavez, who was fluent in Spanish and an excellent teacher. Later, another fine teacher, Sister Elise Horihan, joined the group.

Working with the rector and faculty of the Catholic University of Peru, Franciscans created a university center for Sisters, Regina Mundi. The center offered classes from leading professors toward an Associate of Arts (AA)

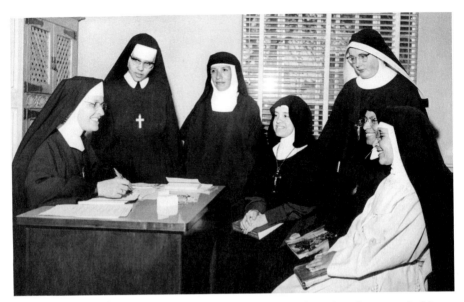

Sister Gretchen Berg and Franciscan colleagues established a university center in Lima, Peru, to help native Sisters raise their level of education. (From Assisi Heights Archives.)

degree. After receiving the AA degree, Sisters were eligible for the university's Bachelor of Arts program. "The success of *Regina Mundi*," Sister Gretchen recalled, "depended on the endorsement of major superiors and novice directors. I began visiting congregational motherhouses across the city of Lima. Meeting with Sisters in their homes gave me a valuable perspective and helped establish relationships. In time, young Sisters from a variety of congregations enrolled in the *Regina Mundi* program.

"Fortunately, my years in Peru, from 1963 to 1967, paralleled the Second Vatican Council. Latin American bishops and theologians were key players at the Council and Peruvians followed the Council closely. At *Regina Mundi*, we designed a three-year Council Renewal Program for major superiors and novice directors. We were delighted when 90 Sisters joined the program. By design, our program began about the same time that the Council ended. The documents of Vatican II, which promulgated decisions on 16 major topics, were literally rolling off the presses. The documents were our textbooks. Topics ranged from lay leadership to ecumenism and renewal of religious life. Three priest theologians, just back from the Council, offered lectures from first-hand experience. Our Sister participants studied the documents, listened to lectures, and implemented renewal in their congregations." Sister Gretchen paused and gave a dazzling smile, "I can tell you—it was exciting!"

In 1967, Mother Callista asked Sister Gretchen to return to Rochester. Elected congregational president 4 years later, Sister Gretchen did not forget her Peruvian experience. "I learned *that* in Peru," she often said. Sister Gretchen referred to the human values she and other Franciscans in Latin America grew to appreciate more deeply, among them, the dignity of each person, the transforming power of relationships, and the importance of personal decisions. As a spiritual leader in a period of enormous change, the values she proclaimed made a significant impact. The congregation's ground-breaking document, the *Philosophy of Sponsorship*, conceived under her leadership, would have far-reaching consequences for Saint Marys Hospital.

In 1967, Sister Consuelo (Marguerite) volunteered to work with American missionaries in the Diocese of Chulucanas, located in the mountains of northern Peru. Rochester Franciscans soon joined her. "I was blessed to be able to work in Peru for 21 years," Sister Ruth Snyder commented. "One of the reasons it was such a rich experience was that the Diocese of Chulucanas had a Pastoral Plan. That meant that everything we did, whether that was catechesis, religious formation, teacher training, social programs, health care, or leadership development, was part of reaching that pastoral goal."

"We had to be adaptable," Sister Ruth also noted. Sisters traveled to the diocese's 1,400 mountain villages by foot, donkey, mule, bicycle, or jeep, whatever was available. Further, they lived entirely on donations from the church, family, and friends. Three Sisters from Saint Marys also volunteered to serve in Chulucanas: Sisters Dora Medina (Juan), Elizabeth (Maristella) Gillis, and Mary Ann Dols. After 20 years as nursing supervisor in obstetrics at Saint Marys Hospital, Sister Dora spent 15 years in Chulucanas endearing herself to everyone who knew her. Sister Patricia "Pat" Himmer, who currently serves Mayo patients at the Gift of Life Transplant House, also ministered in Chulucanas for over 10 years. "It was an immersion experience in a culture much different from our own," Sister Pat recalled. "We lived with the eyes and hearts of a people who struggled for food and survival, yet showed unlimited hospitality, great simplicity, and never tired of learning."

The Latin American opportunity to work with the poor captured the idealism of Franciscans in the States. Sisters admired, and some would emulate, these women who generously served the poor at considerable cost to themselves. Later, when they could choose their own ministries,

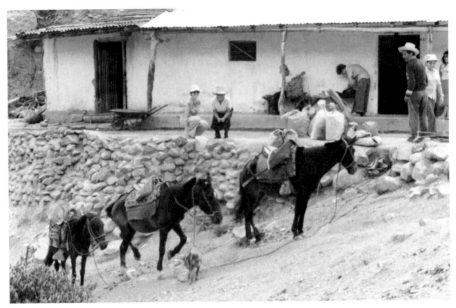

As missionaries in the mountains of northern Peru, Franciscans used whatever trans-
portation was available, including donkeys, to reach the mountain villages they served.
(From Assisi Heights Archives.)

many Sisters left congregational institutions and schools to work with
the poor in the United States and abroad. At Saint Marys, the number of
Sisters who left hospital positions for these ministries had a major impact
on the institution.

Like their counterparts at Saint Marys Hospital, 180,000 American Sisters
looked with hope to the Second Vatican Council. "They had labored for
more than a century to build the American Catholic Church into a most
remarkable institution," writes John J. Fialka. "Now the sisters were looking
for signs of respect from within the Church and a fairer, more equal voice
in its governance. Their case was a good one. Their schools, universities,
and hospitals were thriving. The number of women entering convents was
nearing an all-time high."

A small book, published as the Council opened, created a major impact.
The Nun in the World animated critical discussion among Sisters about reli-
gious life, perhaps for the first time. The author, Belgian Cardinal Joseph
Suenens, was a close friend of John XXIII. *The Nun in the World*, writes
Kenneth A. Briggs, "was nothing less than a brief for sweeping change."
An advance excerpt "took many Catholics by storm. Publication of the entire

book only broadened and sharpened the debate." Pointedly, the book's caption reads, "The Cardinal poses no revolution . . . unless it be revolutionary to attempt to guide toward a concerted effort the immense potential of 1,000,000 nuns."

Cardinal Suenens' description of nuns resonated with many Franciscans. "She appears to the faithful to be out of touch with the world as it is: an anachronism. She is too isolated, too remote, too encased in a habit that estranges her from the very people she would serve, some of whom associate her with a certain childishness, a naiveté." In his opinion, Sisters let sexism in society and the church intimidate them. "The antifeminist tradition has had a long inning . . . As a nun she will not allow herself to claim even a few of the rights that women have managed to obtain bit by bit from man in our modern society." Urging Sisters to free themselves from "the minutiae of canon law," Cardinal Suenens advocated reform in dress, living arrangements, and working conditions.

Sadly, Sisters' high expectations for religious renewal and clerical respect ebbed with the hard realities of Vatican II. "Nuns stood at the periphery as the conclave was planned and started," notes Briggs. "Sisters and women in general were excluded from the commissions preparing the agenda and from the official invitees. Neither their views nor their counsel was sought in any significant way." When Cardinal Suenens reminded the Council that Vatican II failed to represent "half of humanity," few seemed to hear. At the final session, 15 Sisters were permitted to sit in the third balcony of St. Peter's. Far below them were the 2,500 clerical men who alone debated the issues, drafted the documents, and defined the outcomes of the Second Vatican Council.

The Vatican document, *Perfectae Caritatis*, "The Decree on the Renewal of Religious Life," was directed to religious. Unfortunately, Sisters had no voice in writing the document, nor did they review it before publication. Vaguely written, *Perfectae Caritatis* was approved in the rush of the Council's final days. "On its face, the document lacked vigor, clarity," notes Briggs. "But its implications were profound, even revolutionary to the degree that they seemed to authorize a wholesale redesign of the sisterhood." *Perfectae Caritatis* recommended the adaptation of lifestyles to changing social conditions. Further, it authorized experimentation with the approval of the General Chapter, the congregation's highest governing body. Permanent changes required a formal petition to Rome and extensive examination by Vatican canon lawyers.

Franciscans addressed *Perfectae Caritatis* and the Council documents in congregational meetings. With the Gospels as a foundation, Sisters studied the literature, listened to presentations, and discussed issues in small groups. Discussions flowed reasonably well on abstract issues. Requests for experimentation in dress, ministry, and community living triggered strong differences. In general, women who joined the congregation during and after World War II favored change in varying degrees. Others, if not opposed to change, were cautious and less invested. Still others objected to change entirely. When the 1968 General Chapter convened at Assisi Heights, experimentation went forward, though not without lengthy discussion and serious objections.

For the first time Sisters could decide what they wore, where they worked, and with whom they lived. A new interpretation of the vow of obedience ended the traditional practice of assigning Sisters to congregational schools and institutions. A number of Franciscans, who continued to work at Saint Marys moved to small houses and apartments in the area. Still others left the hospital entirely to serve in new ministries. Within a period of 3 years, 20 head nurses, all of them Sisters, left Saint Marys Hospital.

In the early 1970s, Sister Florence Zweber, assistant administrator for Fiscal Affairs and Systems Management, left Saint Marys Hospital for a position at Seattle University. Later, in response to an appeal for health care workers, Sister Florence joined the United Farm Workers (UFW) as a nurse in 1976. When UFW leader Cesar Chavez learned about Sister Florence's financial management background, he appointed her head of the union's accounting department. Larry Albrecht, who visited Sister Florence at UFW headquarters, recalled, "She did a similar administrative and financial overhaul for the migrant farm workers' system as she had at Saint Marys." Sister Florence was named to UFW's board of directors and helped with schools of collective bargaining. Tragically, Sister Florence was killed in a car accident in Tahachapi, California, in 1981. Cesar Chavez, who came to Rochester for her funeral, confided, "If there was a question I could ask of Sister Florence it would be this: 'how will the United Farm Workers get along without you?'"

In 1971, Sister Jean Keniry took a nursing position with the National Farm Workers Service Center in Mission, Texas. During her years in Texas, she studied at Texas Women's University in Houston, where she earned a masters degree in Community Nursing. In 1976, at the request of Sister Kathleen Van Groll, now president of the congregation, she returned to

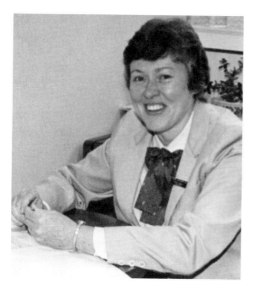

Sister Jean Keniry was appointed Saint Marys Hospital's director of nursing in 1978. (From Saint Marys Hospital Archives.)

Saint Marys Hospital as associate director of nursing. Two years later, Sister Jean was named director of nursing. Recalling those years in south Texas, "It was a life-changing experience, completely different from anything I'd known," she said. "The culture, the people, health-care issues, even the climate were new learning opportunities for me. I gained a great deal personally and professionally."

Quiet and self-effacing, Sister Philothea Kadrlik, the hospital convent's housekeeper, found a new opportunity right at Saint Marys Hospital. When Sister Philothea became a Franciscan in 1935, two of her siblings were already congregational housekeepers, Sisters Julia and Agnes Kadrlik. The Kadrliks, hard-working farmers of Czech background, had 12 children. "I liked school," recalled Sister Philothea, "but our parents couldn't afford to send us beyond eighth grade. Even so, I continued to read a good deal. When I went to Saint Marys Hospital, I enjoyed the staff library. Sister Geralda Costello was the librarian, a wonderful person; I helped her shelve books whenever I could. In 1971, I learned about an opening for an 'assistant to the assistant librarian.' I had always wanted to work in a library. I asked for an interview and got the job! Sister Geralda was patient and I learned a good deal. When she retired, her replacement gave me many more new tasks. By the time I retired, I knew almost enough to run the library!"

A number of hospital Sisters chose to leave religious life entirely. Their decisions

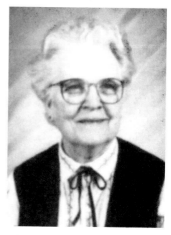

Sister Philothea Kadrlik realized a life-long goal when she became an assistant librarian. (Courtesy of Sister Philothea Kadrlik.)

were deeply personal and often painful. For some, the strain of prolonged service in surgery and acute care areas figured in the decision. A former member later shared, "Even after I was hospitalized for exhaustion, there was no relief. Since eighth grade I wanted to be a Sister, but I couldn't live like that, physically, emotionally, or spiritually." Sister Gretchen Berg was president of the congregation at the time many Sisters left. "For me, thank God, it was a time of unusual grace. When I met with these beautiful young women, a sense of quiet within allowed me to hear their stories. They made vows with every intention of staying in the congregation for life. This wasn't going to happen—they were with us only for a time. Yet I believed they would make a greater contribution when they left for having this experience. And, of course, we gained immeasurably from having them with us."

The Sisters who chose to remain at Saint Marys Hospital experienced profound loss and painful adjustment. Shifting patterns of community living and the departures of friends and colleagues were daily realities. They often supervised employees who questioned why Sisters left their responsibilities. Many employees felt deeply disappointed, even betrayed, by the loss of Sisters they had known for years. "The decade was one of uncertainty and sadness, anger and bewilderment, discovery and hope," notes the hospital's centennial history. "The community resembled a family and now the family was breaking up . . . the Sisters rarely spoke openly about the changes and those who were leaving. It was too painful." Nevertheless, the Franciscans' highest priority remained the welfare of each patient, sometimes at heroic cost.

Sister Mary Lou Connelly never doubted her own decision to remain at the hospital. "Saint Marys was our hospital, our home, we owned it, and it was our responsibility," she said. "Patients trusted us to give them the best care in the world." An instructor in Saint Marys School of Nursing, Sister Mary Lou was part of another difficult change when the diploma school closed in 1970. Founded in 1906 by Sister Joseph Dempsey, the 3-year nursing program had a history of remarkable achievement. Nursing schools increasingly affiliated with collegiate programs for a broader academic background. In the mid 1960s Saint Marys Hospital and Rochester Methodist Hospital agreed to close their diploma programs "with certain conditions." "At this time," writes Virginia Simons Wentzel, "80% of nursing needs in the country was still being met by diploma graduates. There could be no abrupt cut off of this supply of nursing." The Rochester State Junior College developed a 2-year associate degree nursing program in collaboration with the hospitals. Students continued to have clinical experiences at both hospitals. Almost 900 alumni attended the 1970 closing of Saint Marys School of Nursing. In her final address, Sister Mary Brigh Cassidy, class of '27, recalled the school's traditions and the alumni's contribution to nursing care. Her quiet words in conclusion spoke to the hearts of all assembled, "It has been so good."

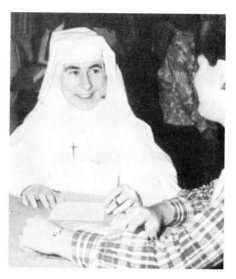

The closing of diploma schools highlighted the country's serious shortage of nurses. A dramatic increase in the demand for health care made the shortage a national concern. Several factors accounted for the growing demand, Medicare

Sister Mary Lou Connelly taught nursing to students in Saint Marys School of Nursing and Saint Marys School of Practical Nursing. (From Saint Marys Hospital Bulletin, September 1965.)

foremost among them. Widely subscribed prepaid insurance plans also removed financial barriers to seeking medical care. Powerful third parties, government, Medicare, and insurance companies, began to exert a new and powerful impact on health care institutions.

Saint Marys Hospital, like its national counterparts, moved to a new era during the late 1960s. With this shift, Sister Mary Brigh took bold initiatives to ensure the hospital's growth and stability. With the numbers of Sisters declining, she looked to the laity for hospital leadership. The Vatican Council's proclamations on the laity probably influenced her decision; at the least, it legitimized her direction. Moreover, Sister Mary Brigh had entered religious life as a professional woman at the age of 30. Her positive experiences working with lay colleagues affirmed her present decision. She valued the broad perspective of lay colleagues and respected their judgment.

On July 31, 1968, Saint Marys Hospital was incorporated as a legal entity separate from the congregation and placed under the direction of a board of trustees. Fifteen persons comprised the Board, seven laypersons and eight Franciscans. Lay members provided a new and valuable dimension of oversight and advice. "Saint Marys was no longer a service involving

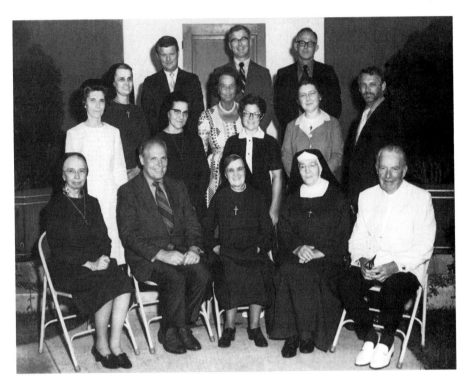

Sister Mary Brigh established the Saint Marys Board of Trustees in 1968. Pictured above is the first board of trustees. Front row (left to right): Sister Mary Brigh Cassidy, Mr. Ray L. Roberts, Sister Adele O'Neil, Mother Callista Hynes, Mr. James J. Thornton. Middle row (left to right): Sister Florence Zweber, Sister Generose Gervais, Sister Millicent Kuechenmeister, Mrs. Howard K. Gray, Sister Kateri Heckathorn, Sister Alcantra Schneider, Mr. Thomas E. Wolf. Back row (left to right): Mr. Robert S. Brown, Mr. David A. Leonard, George W. Morrow, Jr., M.D. (From Saint Marys Hospital Archives.)

only the patient and the hospital," commented David A. Leonard. "It became important to involve others who were sensitive to third parties and the legislative process to give Saint Marys that added depth."

Dave Leonard, who served 14 years on the board, eight of them as president, recalled his first years as a trustee. "Board membership was a new experience for lay members and Sisters alike. At first, the meetings were extremely polite. Sister Mary Brigh was so accustomed to making her own decisions that the Board became kind of a social function. With the 282 Project, later the Mary Brigh Building, the Board became fully functioning." Physician George W. Morrow, Jr., M.D., businessmen James J. Thornton and Robert S. Brown, banker Ray L. Roberts, attorney Thomas E. Wolf, community leader Mrs. Howard K. Gray, and Mayo administrator David A. Leonard brought valuable perspectives to the board room.

Robert "Bob" Brown, owner of a successful insurance business with his father, was in his mid 30s when Sister Mary Brigh invited him to join the Board. Bob knew Sister Mary Brigh through his parents, notably his mother—they were girlhood friends. "It was an unusual opportunity for a young man," he recalled. "Once in a lifetime you meet someone like Sister Mary Brigh. She had a quiet manner with an extraordinary ability to grasp complex issues and express them clearly. Working with the building committee on the 282 Project, I observed her interactions closely. Sister Mary Brigh held her own with contractors—she was firm but fair. I was on the Board for 15 years. What a great privilege. I'll always be thankful that Sister Mary Brigh asked me to serve."

During the Board's 18-year history, a wide variety of gifted and dedicated trustees, Sisters and laypersons, made incisive decisions on vital issues. Working in small committees, trustees and community representatives focused on particular areas, among them building, finance, personnel, and public affairs. Subsequently, trustees brought committee recommendations to the board for discussion. In 1986, when Saint Marys Hospital, Rochester Methodist, and the Mayo Clinic elected to merge into a single organization, the Saint Marys Hospital Board ended its remarkable history. Dave Leonard considered the significance of the Board of Trustees. "This first sharing by non-Franciscans in trusteeship grew over the years to include increasing numbers of lay people, triggered in part by lessening numbers of Sisters available to act in these roles . . . The merger of the Mayo Clinic and its two affiliated hospitals was, therefore, developed against a background of gradual transition from total Franciscan direction of the life and mission of Saint Marys to one of partnership with the laity."

When Sister Nora Logan resigned as Personnel Director in 1969, Sister Mary Brigh again looked to lay leadership. She chose 27-year-old Roger Wells, recently discharged from the Air Force. Though Roger had a better job offer at St. Lawrence Hospital in Lansing, Michigan, he opted for Saint Marys Hospital. Later he reflected on his choice. "During my interview, Sister Mary Brigh told me, 'Mr. Wells, if you accept this position, we don't expect you to run Personnel the way it was run in the past.' I asked myself, 'How many organizations would let a young 27-year-old create change?' I believed changes were going to happen at Saint Marys Hospital. I wanted to be part of those changes."

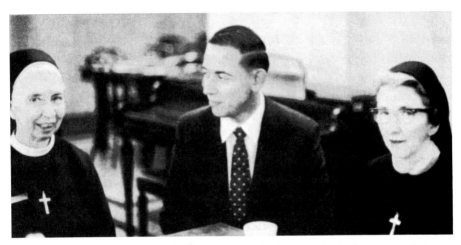

Appointed Personnel Director in 1969, Roger Wells followed in the footsteps of Sister Mary Brigh (left), who initiated the department in 1945, and Sister Nora Logan (right), director from 1947 to 1969. (From Saint Marys Hospital News Bulletin, Vol. XXVII, no. 7, August 1969.)

Over his first 3 years at Saint Marys, Roger hired 30 new managers, all laypersons. His first hire was close to home. "We had only three staff in Personnel," he said, "the director, employment manager Sister Valerie Olson, and our secretary, Margaret Hermann. I requested a second employment manager. When Sister Mary Brigh approved the position, I immediately informed Margaret that she was 'fired.' She was stunned. 'You're the new employment manager,' I hastened to tell her, 'your first assignment is to hire a new secretary.'"

Roger filled existing managerial positions formerly held by Sisters. He also established a number of positions created by technological advances, such as the hospital's new computer system. In the midst of changes and new lay leadership, Roger was touched by the warmth and acceptance of the Sisters. "Franciscans embraced lay people as leaders and showed them mutual respect and hospitality—it was in their bones!"

A headline in the March 1970 *News Bulletin* announced the creation of Department of Pastoral Care. In reality, the function of chaplaincy had been present since the hospital's opening day. Pastors of Saint John the Evangelist, Rochester's first Catholic Church, attended the needs of Saint Marys Hospital. Pioneer pastors, such as Father William Reardon and Father Thomas O'Gorman, served patients, staff, students, and Sisters at Saint Marys for over 40 years. Protestant chaplains also served with great dedication.

Assigned by their churches, they cared for patients at Saint Marys, downtown hospitals, and the Clinic.

Father Raymond Galligan, the first chaplain assigned to Saint Marys, served from 1930 to 1954. Father Galligan visited Catholic patients on every floor three times each day. Reliable as clockwork, he almost sprinted as he arrived in the room. "My name is Galligan," he would say, "How are things going today?" At the time, patients were hospitalized for longer periods, which probably accounts for Father Galligan's relatively short visits. In any case, as *A Century of Caring* notes, "he had time to convey to patients that he cared, and, more importantly, that God cared."

Fathers Daniel Corcoran and Lawrence Murtagh, and other chaplains who served in the 1950s and 1960s, introduced liturgical reforms to the hospital community. Reform brought changes to long-standing religious practices; many Catholics, including Sisters, had difficulty accepting the changes. Nevertheless, the priests persisted. "They got us through Vatican II," commented Jane Campion with a wry smile. In addition to chaplain responsibilities, priests taught religion classes in Saint Marys School of Nursing. Fifty years later, students well remember Father Dan Corcoran and the other chaplains. One graduate recalled that Father Corcoran's comments made a deep impression. Another former student remembered him as a trusted confidant and advocate, "particularly when I got in trouble for something I did!"

The Second Vatican Council's initiatives on ecumenism and lay ministry had a significant influence on the new Pastoral Care Department. Headed by Father Virgil Duellman, the department included 13 chaplains of Catholic, Protestant, and Jewish denominations. Franciscan Sisters JoAnne Lawson, Shane Curran, and Bona Mueller served as Pastoral Associates. In 1973, the department initiated a summer program in Clinical Pastoral Education (CPE) for seminarians. Pastoral Care was fortunate when Darlene Wilson joined the staff as department secretary in 1976. Darlene, who continues to be a welcoming, strengthening presence, commented on her years in Pastoral Care. "Helping patients, families, and staff get the spiritual care they need is a privilege. Being able to help people is one of the richest and rewarding aspects of my career. It's a blessing to be part of this department."

The Sister Visitors program, founded in 1966, served Saint Marys patients under the direction of Sister Antoine Murphy. The March 1970 *News Bulletin* noted, "The 11 Sisters involved in this endeavor strive to make visits at least twice a week. The Sisters are available to perform small courtesies for patients

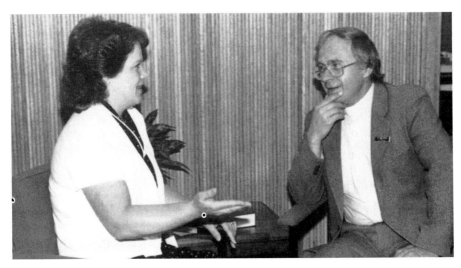

Darlene Wilson and Father James Buryska, of the Department of Chaplain Services, discuss a current department issue. (From Caring, Summer 1987, p 3.)

and their families, to assist distressed or bereaved families, and to expedite the work of chaplains." Lynn Frederick, the current administrator of Saint Marys Hospital, noted the continued contribution of Franciscans who reside at the hospital. "For patients and families the opportunity to meet the Sisters is very important. Whether as Sister Visitors or volunteering in another way, patients are deeply grateful to Sisters for making themselves available. The Franciscans' presence at Saint Marys is a gift to all of us, patients, families, and staff."

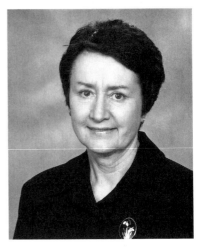

Lynn Frederick currently serves as administrator of Saint Marys Hospital. (From Mayo Clinic Archives.)

When Father Duellman left as director of the department in 1977, Sister Generose asked Sister Helen Hayes to take the position. Sister Helen, then serving in parish retreat ministry, returned to Saint Marys. Father James Buryska recalled Sister Helen's contribution. "She was a highly qualified professional herself, and she expected this level of expertise and practice from her colleagues. To broaden the department, she hired the hospital's first non-Roman Catholic chaplain, Barry O'Brien, a Lutheran pastor. Barry became the new "Protestant Coordinator." Rochester Methodist Hospital had a CPE program that was "state of the art." Sister Helen initiated regular meetings with the director and his staff to learn more about CPE. She raised the standards of the Saint Marys program and broadened participation to include women and men of all faiths.

Jane Campion worked closely with Sister Helen. "Helen was a visionary, who implemented the Ecumenical teachings of Vatican II. She took Chaplaincy out of the Catholic culture and developed new models for expanding services to Protestants and Catholics." A new Clinical Pastoral Extended Program, directed by Sister JoAnne Lawson, was characteristic of Sister Helen's initiatives. The 10-week program, explained Sister JoAnne, "helps laypersons raise their levels of awareness to the needs of the sick and develop skills in meeting these needs."

Father Joseph Keefe, who joined the department a year after Sister Helen in 1978, spoke about his experience as a chaplain. "When I came to Pastoral Care, priests distributed Communion to all the patients. Vatican II taught us that Baptism, not Holy Orders, was the most important sacrament. I took the initiative and asked laypersons to help distribute Communion. Some of them, now called Eucharistic Ministers, have continued to serve—they often thank me for this privilege. Chaplaincy was an awakening for me. When I visited patients, I learned to let them stay with their stories rather than hold forth with my opinions. For patients, the experience of telling their stories to an accepting person was therapeutic. They freed themselves of burdens as they talked through their fears, guilt, and other feelings . . . I valued my relationships with staff and learned to listen to them as well," Father Joe continued. "I hope I was helpful to them; I'm grateful for the ways they enriched my life and expanded my vision."

After four decades of service, two of them as hospital administrator, Sister Mary Brigh announced her retirement in 1971. Sister Mary Brigh continued to share her wisdom with the hospital during her retirement years and found more time for writing poetry, an avocation she cherished but had little time to do. Reflecting on her life, she wrote, "Not a particularly courageous person, I grew in self-confidence and courage to take on difficult responsibilities because I knew that was the work God wanted me to do and that He would help me find the right answer, the needed assistance, often in places I would not have expected them." In *Century of Caring's* final tribute, "Although Alzheimer's disease finally stole from Sister Mary Brigh's mind its consistent brilliance, it could not dim the memory of her many accomplishments."

With Sister Mary Brigh's retirement, Sister Generose Gervais was appointed hospital administrator. Accounts of Sister Generose in earlier chapters testify to her remarkable abilities and selfless commitment. Even so, as colleague Marianne Hockema observed, "Perhaps the most important thing to know about Sister Generose Gervais is how easy it is to underestimate her. When you first meet her, she is apt to engage you in a lively conversation . . . about baking bread or canning pickles or combining soybeans. You'd find her to be warm, down-to-earth and intensely practical. You'd probably walk away thinking you'd had a nice visit with a fairly typical woman from southeastern Minnesota who still had strong rural ties."

Roger Wells recalls, "Sister Generose was a legend at the University of Minnesota. Twenty years after she studied for a Masters in Health Administration program, she was still the only student with straight A's!" In those years Sister Generose was often the only woman in the class; she commented on this later in her characteristically direct manner. "Being in class around men didn't bother me because anywhere I was working, I had to work with men. I never thought I was an outcast or looked down on as an inferior . . . I think they always respected me as a woman and a Sister. I didn't expect any privileges because I was a woman and I didn't get any."

When Sister Generose returned from graduate school in 1954, she was appointed assistant administrator to Sister Mary Brigh. Over the next 17 years, as previous chapters note, she had a variety of supervisory projects throughout the hospital. By 1971, *A Century of Caring* notes "she had learned every aspect of the Saint Marys operation." Sister Generose played a crucial role in planning for the new Mary Brigh Building. "Her insistence on economy and accountability kept Saint Marys financially strong during an era in which rising costs drained the coffers of many hospitals." The respect she gained from these accomplishments was not lost on observers. Among her many awards and appointments, Sister Generose was the first woman to serve as a member of the board of directors of the Federal Reserve Bank of Minneapolis.

One of Sister Generose's memorable contributions, and probably among the most rewarding, is the Poverello Foundation. The foundation has at its purpose "to ease the burden for patients who need financial support for the care they received at Saint Marys Hospital." Named for Saint Francis of Assisi, referred to as "Il Poverello" or "the little poor man," the foundation helps about 350 to 400 persons each year. Donations abound from former patients as well as employees. Sister Generose, Sister Lauren Weinandt, and other Sisters at Saint Marys Hospital work to actively raise money for the Poverello Fund. An annual Sisters' bazaar, featuring Sister Generose's jams, jellies, and pickles, raises thousands of dollars. Sister Lauren finds many ways to help the foundation, among them, periodic rummage sales where she and her team of dedicated volunteers, who are retired Saint Marys employees, sell donated items from furniture to toys.

In 1981, the Board of Trustees appointed Sister Generose to the newly created position of Executive Director. Michael Myers, a lawyer and administrator of Catholic hospitals, was named Administrator of Saint Marys Hospital. For the first time in the hospital's history a Franciscan did not head Saint Marys Hospital. Almost a decade earlier, thanks to the initiative of Sister Kathleen Van Groll, the Sisters took steps in anticipation of this change. Sister Kathleen, then assistant hospital administrator, was also congregational vice president under Sister Gretchen Berg. "At her suggestion," notes Sister Patricia Fritz, "the 1973 General Chapter approved a *Philosophy of Sponsorship*. The purpose of the document was to articulate the operative values of an institution sponsored by the Rochester Franciscans." The dignity of each person and the transforming power of relationships were the document's central themes.

In 1986, Mayo Clinic and the two hospitals elected to merge into a single organization. A variety of factors prompted the merger, notes Dave Leonard, "but largely because federal government reimbursement mechanisms made the proper allocation of aggregated payments to the three organizations difficult." Mayo Clinic physicians wanted Franciscan sponsorship to continue: "We know who we are with the Sisters," said W. Eugene Mayberry, M.D., vice-chairman of Mayo Foundation at the time of the merger. "But we don't know who we'd be without them."

With the Sisters' approval, Sister Patricia Fritz, then congregational president, applied her considerable gifts to continue Franciscan sponsorship of Saint Marys as a Catholic hospital. Achieving this objective was not without formidable obstacles. No precedent then existed for Catholic sponsorship of a hospital owned and operated by a secular institution; furthermore, powerful leaders within the Catholic Church opposed setting such a radical precedent. Undaunted, Sister Patricia, assisted by Sister Meigan Fogarty, worked tenaciously for a viable solution. Sister June Kaiser, president of the board of trustees, and the trustees offered counsel and support.

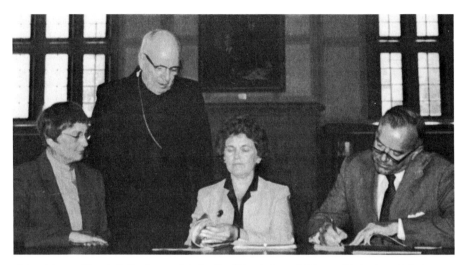

Saint Marys Hospital, Rochester Methodist Hospital, and Mayo Clinic signed their agreement to integrate operations under Mayo Foundation for Medical Education and Research on May 28, 1986. Pictured at the formal signing event, from left are Sister June Kaiser, president of the Saint Marys Board of Trustees; Bishop Loras Watters, Diocese of Winona; Sister Patricia Fritz, president of the Sisters of Saint Francis; and W. Eugene Mayberry, M.D., vice-chairman of Mayo Foundation. (From A Century of Caring: 1889-1989. Rochester, MN: Saint Marys Hospital, 1988, p 109.)

Throughout this period, Sisters Patricia and Meigan consulted with Bishop Loras Watters of the Diocese of Winona and other church leaders. Ultimately, the Sisters redefined the sponsoring role. "Authentic Sponsorship means influencing the environment of the institution, its philosophy, mission, role, and goals." Bishop Watters and the Vatican approved the concept of "Sponsorship by influence" as warranting continued recognition of Saint Marys as a Catholic hospital.

Created as part of the merger, the Saint Marys Hospital Sponsorship Board received an endowment to fund its primary mission: "to preserve the Catholic identity of the hospital and to perpetuate the Mayo/Franciscan values throughout the Rochester campus. In her article for the *St. Anthony Messenger* on the Franciscan roots of Mayo Clinic, Marion Amberg described the Sponsorship Board: "Composed of Franciscan Sisters and lay colleagues, the Sponsorship Board has a far-reaching mission statement. Sponsorship seeks to strengthen the spiritual dimension within the Mayo Clinic; reinforce trust among staff and the anticipation of trustworthiness by patients and their families; and nurture the Mayo/Franciscan values of primacy of the patient, trust, commitment to excellence through teamwork, spiritual support and compassion/respect for those served and serving."

Currently administrator for Franciscan Sponsorship, Sister Mary Eliot Crowley has been associated with the Sponsorship mission since the merger in 1986. "While we don't own or operate the hospital, we do influence the way health care is provided," Sister Mary Eliot is quoted in the *St. Anthony Messenger*, adding that Sponsorship is even more important today than it was in 1986. "Until recent years, most new staff members were familiar with the spiritual roots and background of Mayo Clinic. Mayo Rochester today has more than 29,000 employees including researchers, scientists and doctors from around the world, of all faiths and cultures."

Sister Meigan Fogarty, the first President of the Sponsorship Board, spoke to the purpose of Sponsorship in 1988. "What sponsorship really does is challenge us to look at where we've been as a hospital and where we're going, keeping yesterday alive with the aspirations of tomorrow." Fifteen years later, Sheila Jowsey, M.D., a board member, put it this way. "Sponsorship is the institutional memory of Mayo/Franciscan values—it's Mayo's secret sauce. Sponsorship's task is similar to an Olympic runner who passes the baton to others and they in turn, pass it to the next generation."

Generations of Franciscans and Mayo colleagues continued the legacy that began in 1889 when a group of Franciscan Sisters and a family of doctors built and staffed a hospital in a cornfield. This story, which told the tale of

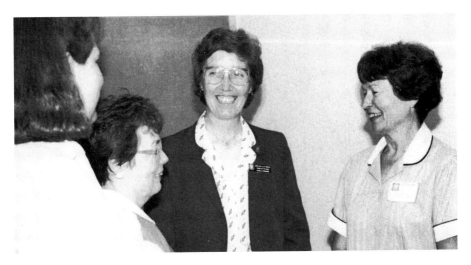

Sister Mary Eliot Crowley currently serves as administrator for Franciscan Sponsorship. (From Caring, Summer 1989, p 23.)

that partnership, described the challenges they faced. Though the challenges were unique for their time, the impetus to overcome them did not vary. Each generation of partners shared a common goal, the welfare of the patient. Inspired by this goal and the dedication they witnessed in each other, generations of Franciscans and Mayo colleagues overcame formidable obstacles. The miracle of healing that happened in past generations does not end; a new generation of Mayo colleagues, inspired with the same purpose, continues to meet the challenges of today through the miracle of relationships.

ENDNOTES

Page 199
     US History—The Peace Corps. **Available from: http://www.peacecorpsonline.org.**

     TIME Man of the Year: Pope John XXIII. **Available from: http://www.time.com. January 4, 1963.**

Pages 199-200
     Bellitto CM: *Renewing Christianity: A History of Church Reform From Day One to Vatican II.* **New York: Paulist Press, 2001, pp 203-204.**

Page 201
     A Century of Caring: 1889-1989. **Rochester, MN: Saint Marys Hospital, 1988, p 88.**

     Interview with Sister Theresa Hoffmann, February 9, 2007.

     Saint Marys Hospital News Bulletin **February 1962.**

Pages 201-202
     Interview with Sister Tierney Trueman, April 4, 2007.

Page 202
     Saint Marys Hospital News Bulletin **August 1963.**

Pages 202-203
     Interview with Sister Jean Schulte, February 13, 2007.

Pages 203-204
     Interview with Sister Gretchen Berg, January 17, 2007.

Page 205
     Interview with Sister Ruth Snyder, February 7, 2007.

     Interview with Sister Patricia Himmer, February 5, 2007.

Page 206
     Fialka JJ: *Sisters: Catholic Nuns and the Making of America.* **New York: St. Martin's Press, 2003, pp 199-200.**

     Briggs KA: *Double Crossed: Uncovering the Catholic Church's Betrayal of American Nuns.* **New York: Doubleday, 2006, p 69.**

Pages 206-207
     Suenens LJ: *The Nun in the World: New Dimensions in the Modern Apostolate.* **Westminster, MD: Newman Press, 1962, pp 33, 45, 49. Cited in Briggs (pp 69, 70, 237).**

Page 207
     Briggs (pp 70, 75, 76).

Page 208
     Interview with Larry Albrecht, November 24, 2006.

Plosknoka-Doré C, Reilly ML: *A Franciscan Symphony of Courage & Creativity*. Rochester, MN: Sisters of Saint Francis, 1999, pp 24-25.

Pages 208-209   Interview with Sister Jean Keniry, March 7, 2007.

Page 209   Interview with Sister Philothea Kadrlik, July 24, 2006.

Pages 209-210   Confidential interviews.

Page 210   Interview with Sister Gretchen Berg, February 14, 2007.

A Century of Caring: 1889-1989, p 88.

Interview with Sister Mary Lou Connelly, September 5, 2005.

Wentzel VS: *Sincere et Constanter 1906-1970: The Story of Saint Marys School of Nursing*. Rochester, MN: Mayo Foundation for Medical Education and Research, 2006, pp 72, 74.

Pages 211-212   A chat with Dave Leonard. *Caring* Spring 1976, p 12.

Page 212   Interview with David A. Leonard, July 18, 2003.

Page 213   Interview with Robert S. Brown, November 10, 2006.

Leonard DA: *Origins of Sponsorship by Influence*. Available from: http://mayoweb.mayo.edu/sponsorship/documents, p 2.

Roger Wells' memoirs, February 23, 2006.

Page 214   Interview with Roger Wells, February 9, 2006.

Saint Marys Hospital News Bulletin March 1970.

Page 215   *A Century of Caring: 1889-1989* (p 66).

Interview with Jane Campion, March 22, 2006.

Interviews with Therese DeGrood and Mary Becker, March 6, 2007.

Interview with Darlene Wilson, March 7, 2007.

Page 216   Interview with Lynn Frederick, March 6, 2007.

Interview with Father James Buryska, February 15, 2006.

Page 217   Interview with Jane Campion, March 22, 2006.

Clinical-Pastoral Ministry Program raises level of awareness. *Caring* **April 1978, pp 3, 4.**

Interview with Father Joseph Keefe, January 27, 2007.

Chaplancy. *Caring* **Summer 1987, p 2.**

Pages 217-218   *A Century of Caring: 1889-1989*, p 96.

Page 218   **Hockema M:** *The Franciscan Five.* **p 39 (unpublished paper).**

Interview with Roger Wells, February 9, 2006.

Interview with Sister Generose Gervais, January 28, 2000.

A Century of Caring: 1889-1989 (pp 102, 104).

Pages 218-219   *Poverello Foundation.* **Rochester, MN: Mayo Foundation for Medical Education and Research, 2005.**

Page 219   **Fritz P:** *Synopsis of the Need for and Evolution of the Concept of Sponsorship.* **Congregational paper, 2003.**

Leonard DA: *Origins of Sponsorship by Influence.* **Available from: http://mayoweb.mayo.edu/sponsorship/documents, p 2.**

Pages 219-220   Interview with Sister Patricia Fritz, February 15, 2007.

Pages 220-221   **Amberg M: Mayo Clinic: The Franciscan connection.** *St. Anthony Messenger* **October 2006, pp 13, 14, 16.**

Page 221   **Saint Marys Sponsorship Board.** *Caring* **Winter 1988, p 11.**

Interview with Dr. Sheila Jowsey, September 12, 2003.

INDEX

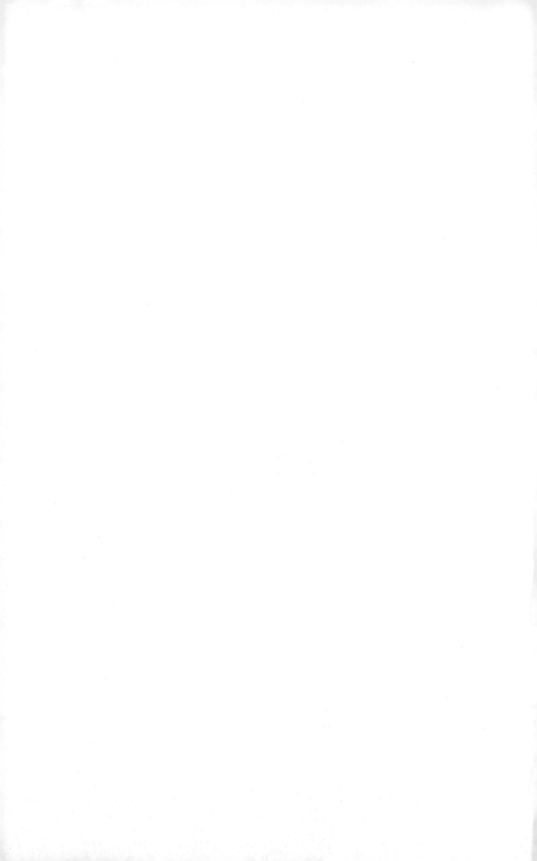